Generalised Predictive Control and Bioengineering

Generalised Predictive Control and Bioengineering

MAHDI MAHFOUF

AND

DEREK A. LINKENS

Department of Automatic Control and Systems Engineering
The University of Sheffield

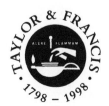

TAYLOR & FRANCIS
ALERE FLAMMAM
1798 – 1998

UK Taylor & Francis Ltd, 1 Gunpowder Square, London EC4A 3DE
USA Taylor & Francis Inc., 1900 Frost Road, Suite 101, Bristol, PA 19007

British Library Cataloguing in Publication Data

A catalogue record for this book is available from the British Library.

ISBN 0-7484-0597-6

Library of Congress Cataloging in Publication data are available

Cover design by Amanda Barragry
Typeset in Times 10/12pt by Santype International Ltd, Salisbury, UK
Printed in Great Britain by T.J. International Ltd, Padstow, UK

Contents

Series Introduction

Control systems has a long and distinguished tradition stretching back to nineteenth-century dynamics and stability theory. Its establishment as a major engineering discipline in the 1950s arose, essentially, from Second World War driven work on frequency response methods by, amongst others, Nyquist, Bode and Wiener. The intervening 40 years has seen quite unparalleled developments in the underlying theory with applications ranging from the ubiquitous PID controller widely encountered in the process industries through to high-performance/fidelity controllers typical of aerospace applications. This development has been increasingly underpinned by the rapid developments in the, essentially enabling, technology of computing software and hardware.

This view of mathematically model-based systems and control as a mature discipline masks relatively new and rapid developments in the general area of robust control. Here intense research effort is being directed to the development of high-performance controllers which (at least) are robust to specified classes of plant uncertainty. One measure of this effort is the fact that, after a relatively short period of work, 'near world' tests of classes of robust controllers have been undertaken in the aerospace industry. Again, this work is supported by computing hardware and software developments, such as the toolboxes available within numerous commercially marketed controller design/simulation packages.

Recently, there has been increasing interest in the use of so-called intelligent control techniques such as fuzzy logic and neural networks. Basically, these rely on learning (in a prescribed manner) the input–output behaviour of the plant to be controlled. Already, it is clear that there is little to be gained by applying these techniques to cases where mature mathematical model-based approaches yield high-performance control. Instead, their role is (in general terms) almost certainly going to lie in areas where the processes encountered are ill-defined, complex, nonlinear, time-varying and stochastic. A detailed evaluation of their (relative) potential awaits the appearance of a rigorous supporting base (underlying theory and implementation architectures for example) the essential elements of which are beginning to appear in learned journals and conferences.

Elements of control and systems theory/engineering are increasingly finding use outside traditional numerical processing environments. One such general area in which there is increasing interest is intelligent command and control systems which are central, for example, to innovative manufacturing and management of advanced transportation systems. Another is discrete event systems which mix numeric and logic decision making.

It was in response to these exciting new developments that the present book series of Systems and Control was conceived. It publishes high-quality research texts and reference works in the diverse areas which systems and control now includes. In addition to basic theory, experimental and/or application studies are welcome, as are expository texts where theory, verification and applications come together to provide a unifying coverage of a particular topic or topics.

E. ROGERS
J. O'REILLY

Acknowledgements

We would like to express our sincere thanks to a number of people and organisations who were instrumental in helping in the research work behind this manuscript. First, we thank Dr A. J. Asbury, a Reader in Anaesthesia at the Glasgow Western Infirmary, for his collaboration and valuable expertise in arranging and helping to conduct most of the clinical trials whose results are presented in this book. His enthusiasm over the years is greatly acknowledged and appreciated. Our thanks are extended to Dr W. M. Gray for his help in making sure that everything was ready prior to going into the operating theatre. We also thank Dr J. E. Peacock, a consultant anaesthetist at the Royal Hallamshire Hospital, for his help in organising some of the trials in Sheffield.

A great proportion of the results presented in this book were obtained while authors were being funded by two Leverhulme Trust Research Grants entitled: 'Design of Generic Intelligent Adaptive Control Architectures Applicable to Anaesthesia' and 'Development of Generic Physiologically-based Models with Application to Anaesthesia'. The help from the trust is gratefully acknowledged.

The authors would also like to thank Dr M. F. Abbod for his help in preparing one of the chapters of this book. Thanks are also extended to past students and research assistants who were part of the same group in the Department of Automatic Control and Systems Engineering, The University of Sheffield, among them Drs M. Menad, M. Khelfa, N. Denai, M. Mansour and E. Tanyi for their friendship over the years. Last, but not least, Mahdi Mahfouf would like to thank his wife, Amanda, for her patience, understanding and support over the years, his parents for the support and love they have unequivocally given him throughout his career, his brothers and sisters as well as their families. Similarly, Derek Linkens wishes to record his thanks to his wife, Ruth, and the extended family for their support and interest over many years in long hours of research into many aspects of biomedical engineering.

MAHDI MAHFOUF AND DEREK A. LINKENS
Sheffield
27 October 1997

CHAPTER ONE

Introduction

Most of the foundations for control and systems theory were laid down by the early 1940s and because of the lack of fast and powerful processing machines to execute their associated algorithms, the majority of the work remained purely theoretical for some time, regardless of whether it was significant or not. It is only in the last three decades that a drastic development of the theory has been witnessed thanks to rapid advances in electronics and particularly computer technology which helped to set up obvious application areas and create new ones, thus making control engineering a discipline of key importance.

The last area of science related to control engineering is clinical medicine which is affected to such an extent that it is now possible to use on-line control devices during surgical operations and even in intensive care units. While this change of attitude towards engineering and particularly control engineering is welcome, it is worth mentioning that safety has been the main catalyst in this progress. Indeed, just as in all other application areas of control engineering like mining, hazardous industry, air travel or nuclear power production, clinical medicine had to be convinced that control is effective and, most importantly, safe. On the one hand safety is very much dependent on how reliable the electronic equipment, that is monitoring devices, computers, etc. is, and parallel advances in technology have helped to establish exactly that. On the other hand, the effective contribution of control is a factor which depends on theoretical results as well as real-time experiments; in other words, safety and effectiveness go hand in hand.

Current application areas of control engineering in clinical medicine constitute a wide spectrum ranging from simple dosage prescriptions to highly sophisticated controllers able to perform more complex tasks such as the control of depth of anaesthesia via a multiple drug infusion system. However, it must be stressed that in all cases the physician forms an integral part of any devised control loop and thus control engineering thrives in playing an assistant role for the physician rather than the substitute role in decision-making or in the execution of his decisions, thus freeing him for more demanding human tasks which no computer can ever accomplish.

This book is mainly devoted to the use of one particular control technique in clinical medicine and represents work which emanates from a period of research which spans more than seven years. Several factors have helped to consolidate this initiative:

1. The international interest that the work on control applications in biomedicine has generated over the years.

2. A personal interest in the application of engineering methods in biomedicine for over a decade.

3. The challenging nature of the discipline which makes almost every experiment carried out represent a test case.

4. The way the barrier between the life sciences and engineering has been reduced to make way for a unique partnership between the two which can achieve difficult but realistic objectives.

In the following sections we will introduce the concepts which this work relied upon, and terminology used in this book as well as describe the content of this book.

1.1   Fundamental definitions

- Pharmacology: a science which studies the metabolism of drugs.
- Pharmacokinetics: a branch of pharmacology which studies what the body does to the drug.
- Pharmacodynamics: a branch of pharmacology which studies what the drug does to the body.
- Anaesthesia: it is defined as that part of the medical science profession which ensures that the patient's body remains insensitive to painful surgical stimuli. It comprises muscle relaxation (paralysis), unconsciousness (narcosis), and analgesia (pain relief).

1.2   Automatic control in biomedicine

It was about 30 years ago that the link between the mathematics of control theory and drug treatment strategies was discovered and published (Bluell *et al.*, 1969). Further research (Smolen *et al.*, 1972) confirmed the identity of drug administration and a class of control problems. The formulation of the problem such that computers could be used conveniently in its solution came as a natural consequence (Bellman, 1971; Sheiner *et al.*, 1972). We are not claiming that all clinical problems can be solved using computers, but merely that computers may prove helpful in situations where theory and reality are somewhat close. Although common to all engineering disciplines, control can be split into two classes: open-loop control and closed-loop control.

1.2.1   Open-loop control

The applications of control theory relied mostly on some deterministic assumptions (Bluell *et al.*, 1969; Bellman, 1971) and the general approach adopted in open-loop configurations is to assume that the pharmacokinetic relationships can be modelled *exactly* by a linear system with exactly known parameters. A performance index is chosen (the integral of the error between a set of drug concentration profiles and the simulated profile). This form of control is known as target concentration infusion (TCI), i.e. given only an understanding of the concentration–effect relationship, a target concentration (drug concentration in the blood) is achieved which, on the basis of available information, is most likely to yield a desired effect. In some cases the target is not static as it is continuously evaluated each time the physician learns more about the patient's response to dosing.

General anaesthesia, whose characterisation is not easily quantifiable, is where this form of control has thrived most. Many commercial devices which incorporate an open-loop strategy already exist such as the target concentration infusion system for the anaesthetic drug propofol developed by White and Kenny (1990), or the commercial system Infus O.R. (Bard Ltd) which uses magnetically coded 'smart labels' to facilitate programming and to help eliminate computing errors. The system offers a variety of such cards for commonly used drugs and permits loading doses and infusion schemes to be implemented quickly and easily and without need for calculation. Shafer (1995) has developed a computer program called STAN-PUMP which allows the physician to select a particular drug from a choice of anaesthetic agents as well as analgesics and also to select the parameters associated with the pharmacokinetic relationship of the drug. This gives the physician more flexibility in the controller's choice, although it is open loop.

However, this deterministic approach to dosage optimisation does not take into account the individuality of each patient since the optimisation procedure is based on the average parameters of a population which makes the solution sub-optimal. In subsequent studies the pharmacodynamic effect of the drug was included instead of only drug concentration in the blood (Jacobs and Williams, 1993). Although this was found to reflect better the mechanism of drug/body interaction, the controller performance was reported to be poor outside the anticipated range of parameter tolerances.

1.2.2 Closed-loop control

Closed-loop control in biomedicine has emerged as a serious contender for all forms of control and in the late 1970s the gap which existed between feedback control and continuous infusion of chemical substances necessary for regulating physiological variables (blood pressure, muscle relaxation) was bridged when research work conducted by pioneers in this field such as Sheppard *et al.* (1979) and Asbury *et al.* (1980) proved through clinical experiments on humans as well as animals that this form of control is safe and effective and in many cases better than manual control.

Feedback control methods in clinical medicine can be grouped into two classes: adaptive and non-adaptive.

Non-adaptive control schemes

Figure 1.1 is a diagram representative of simple non-adaptive closed-loop control in which the controller calculates the necessary drug infusion according to an observation of the therapeutic effect but with a physician acting as an overall supervisor ready to override the controller output if necessary. The watchful eye of the physician represents an integral part of any fully automated control system for two reasons:

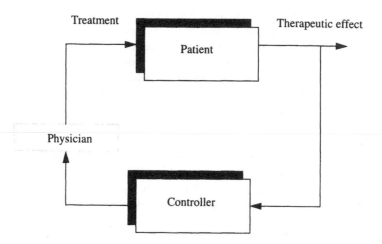

Figure 1.1 Simple closed-loop control scheme.

1. It is often difficult to measure the therapeutic effect at a fast enough sampling rate, especially if it involves painful or harmful procedures such as muscle stimulation or artery squeezing, etc.
2. It is often difficult to model the dose–effect relationships with simple systems.

This has been found to be particularly true in anaesthesia and intensive care medicine where variables are not accessible or cannot even be defined, such as unconsciousness or pain.

The assumption behind non-adaptive control methods or fixed-gain controllers is that the dose–effect relationship can be modelled as a deterministic process with known constant parameters, absurd assumptions since the parameters associated with individual patients are not known.

In cases where parameters remain within acceptable bands of the average parameters (usually obtained from off-line studies), these fixed-gain controllers are known to perform very well providing that the feedback information is rich enough. However, for larger parameter deviations, poor performances should be expected (Chilcoat, 1980; Slate, 1980).

Three-term controllers (that is, proportional, integral and derivative type controllers) are at the forefront of the commonly used type of fixed-gain controllers (Brown *et al.*, 1980; Ebert *et al.*, 1986; Slate *et al.*, 1979). In these applications, offsets coupled with oscillations were recorded and were largely due to the variability of time delay for which there is no information prior to an operation.

Adaptive controllers

Adaptive controllers have been a centre of attention since the late 1980s. Mainly concerned with feedback systems, the term 'adaptive' means that the controller fulfils two tasks at the same time which can be summarised as follows:

1. Controlling the process.
2. Adapting itself to that process and its disturbances in order to achieve satisfactory control.

Therefore, adaptive control can be described as being a generalisation of classical linear feedback control, in the sense that in classical control the coefficients of the law are time-invariant and probably obtained during an off-line study, whereas adaptive control theory produces a controller which tunes itself as the process parameters vary. The associated algorithms are called 'self-tuning algorithms'. The approach was first proposed by Kalman (1958) who made an attempt to implement the algorithm on a computer. A block diagram of a self-tuning control system is shown in Figure 1.2. At each sampling instant the parameters in an assumed dynamic model are estimated recursively from input–output data and the controller settings are then updated. The control design simply accepts current estimates and ignores their uncertainties by evoking the principle of certainty equivalence (Astrom and Wittenmark, 1989; Goodwin and Sin, 1984) which states simply that the self-tuning properties should still hold if the true parameter estimates are replaced by their estimated ones. The principle represents, in fact, the cornerstone of the theory as it facilitated the solving of many practical problems, especially those of a non-linear nature.

Self-tuning controllers can, however, be based on several techniques which although different in structure use the same philosophy, that is regulating around a certain point, be it a single-input single-output (SISO) or a multi-input multi-output (MIMO) situation. Space prohibits mentioning all of them, but Pole-Placement (Wellstead, 1980), general minimum variance (GMV) (Clarke and Gawthrop, 1975, 1979; Gawthrop, 1977) and Generalised Predictive Control (GPC) (Clarke *et al.*,

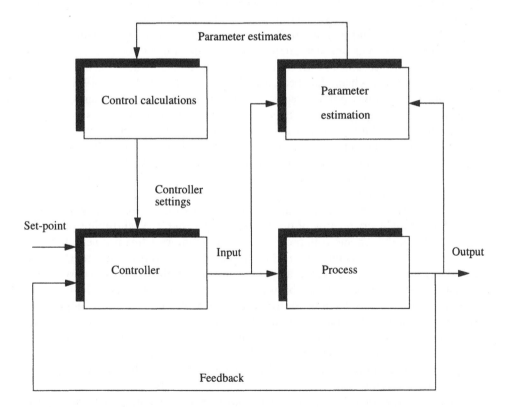

Figure 1.2   Self-tuning control system.

1987a, 1987b) are among the best known algorithms. They mainly fall into two categories: explicit and implicit algorithms. The first category implies that the regulator parameters are updated indirectly via estimation of the process parameters, whereas in the second category, the control design stage is omitted by producing directly the coefficients of the required control law. It is worth noting that most of these techniques are based on a linear model formulation although some of them can and have been extended to nonlinearity structures such as Volterra series, bilinear models, etc.

The use and success of adaptive controllers in biomedicine is due to several factors:

1. The large inter-individual and intra-individual variability of the patient's parameters.

2. The increasing availability of reliable and cheap technology such as monitors and computers.

3. The rapid theoretical development of adaptive control techniques which were backed by strong stability results.

4. The birth of a new era of rapprochement between clinicians who were eager to develop their skills and control engineers who wished to test their designs and see them work.

Of course adaptation to patients' parameter changes can be analysed from two different aspects. The first aspect is that the parameters of the individual are determined prior to surgery via measurements after administration of a unit-dose (impulse response) and the controller tuned exactly for those parameters, this method being known as one-step adaptation. This method is known to be successful if the individual's parameters are not thought to change on-line during an operation. Although this scheme has been used in the past (Tatnall *et al.*, 1981; Salzsieder *et al.*, 1984), it has not proved very popular because measurements prior to surgery are not always possible. The second aspect is that the patient's parameters are identified continuously, based on linear or nonlinear autoregressive models of the dose–effect relationship (Koivo, 1981). The control law, utilising the above self-tuning algorithms, can be calculated from those parameters. Despite their main asset which is the principle of certainty equivalence, and like any feedback control, these controllers require that the input–output information is 'rich enough' (or persistently exciting) to be able to conduct the identification phase successfully, especially during nonlinear regions of operation. Failing that, the self-tuning properties will be lost and the scheme collapses. In order to counteract this problem, the original techniques were amended to include jacketing procedures ready to take over should anything go wrong. Hence, adaptive control with the physician as part of the loop, as shown in Figure 1.3, has been more successful if only to give the physician the opportunity to override any controller output based on his clinical judgment at any time. Similarly to open-loop control, adaptive control laws which are based (either implicitly or explicitly) on an optimisation operation have proved more popular because they take into account the therapeutic effect as well as drug consumption in the cost function to be optimised, parameters which coincide very much with the clinicians' thinking when performing manual control.

Numerous types of self-adaptive scheme have been studied in biomedical applications. These include post-operative blood pressure and muscle relaxant adminis-

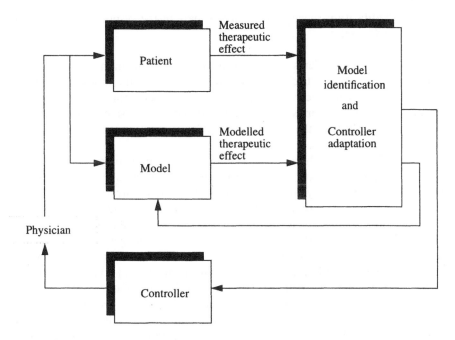

Figure 1.3 Adaptive control scheme in which a model of the patient is continuously updated via an identification algorithm. This, in turn, is used to adapt the controller parameters to give a good control performance (after Vozeh and Steimer, 1985).

tration. Much of the early and later work on blood pressure centred around the key work on identification studies performed by Sheppard and Slate (Slate, 1980; Sheppard, 1983) which revealed dynamic features such as recirculation effect and background activity containing both stochastic and sinusoidal components. Using this model a number of control designs using the drug sodium-nitroprusside (SNP) and mean arterial pressure measurements (MAP) have been undertaken, including adaptive gain control (Koivo, 1980), pole-placement algorithm (Mansour and Linkens, 1988) and long-range adaptive predictive control (Kwok *et al.*, 1995). Using inhalational drugs such as isoflurane, Millard *et al.* (1988a) used the well-known Clarke and Gawthrop algorithm to control blood pressure during surgery. In this case control was maintained via adjustment of the inspired concentration of isoflurane delivered to patients requiring induced hypotension during ENT surgery.

In muscle relaxation, various linear adaptive controllers have been designed for drugs such as pancuronium (Linkens *et al.*, 1985), atracurium (Denai *et al.*, 1990; Linkens *et al.*, 1991). One common challenge characterised the atracurium controller design during the initial phase of muscle relaxation (paralysis) induction. This was that a large dose of muscle relaxant had to be administered to the patient to start surgery promptly, which meant that the paralysis level saturated for a while. As a result, the control loop was not closed until the paralysis level reached a certain level judged to be adequate. This posed two problems:

1. Due to the nonlinear nature of the process, any large control dose can cause the paralysis level to saturate again.

2. The identification scheme misses a key part of the response for identifying the process dynamics.

Solutions to these problems will be outlined in the forthcoming chapters but suffice to say that a number of 'tricks' used in other disciplines are impossible to reproduce in biomedicine where every experiment is a real experiment as such. Hence, extensive and sometimes pessimistic simulations are conducted to ensure that once transferred to the theatre the controller will perform to everyone's expectations, especially the physician's.

Among the features characterising biomedical systems, time delay is perhaps the most challenging one. The time taken by the drug to circulate around the body is one cause of such a delay, and variation of the cardiac output (the volume of blood pumped by the heart within a unit-time) is another cause. Designing controllers to overcome time delays has always presented a serious challenge for engineers from almost all walks of life. Also this challenge grows even bigger when the value of this time delay is unknown or is prone to variations. PID controllers, whose benefits are still greatly utilised within industry, can prove ineffective in trying to overcome this problem. Indeed, despite their derivative action they are often unable to provide the right phase advance needed and consequently require *retuning* in order to encompass such variations. This operation requires considerable trial and error efforts which can be tiresome and very time consuming. The method of O. J. M. Smith known as the 'Smith Predictor' (Smith, 1959) has been shown to be very advantageous, however its performance may deteriorate considerably in the presence of a large process mismatch, which has led industry to prefer the manually tuned classical PID networks which do not involve the derivation of realistic dynamic process models. This mismatch problem has always been one of the major topics for those who have been involved with time delay systems (Marshall, 1979; Gawthrop, 1977) and the advances achieved in computer technology in the 1970s allowed self-tuning adaptive control, whose origin goes back to the 1950s (Gregory, 1959), to emerge as another alternative for such a problem.

Early well-known self-tuning adaptive algorithms included the minimum variance (MV) controller (Astrom and Wittenmark, 1973), the generalised minimum variance (GMV) with its refined version developed by Clarke and Gawthrop, and the pole-placement algorithm. Over the years these methods proved to be far superior to the classical PID controllers providing the model order as well as the corresponding dead-time value are carefully selected. Indeed, the MV controller showed high sensitivity to a wrongly assumed or variable value of time delay, whereas the improved version of Clarke and Gawthrop (GMV) is somewhat more robust providing it is correctly detuned. Practical work also showed that the pole-placement approach is robust against this assumption (the delay value is enhanced within the numerator polynomial of the discrete-time transfer function), but over-parameterisation often leads to common factors in the estimated polynomials resulting in deterioration of the controller performance.

Since the emergence of self-tuning adaptive techniques as a powerful tool for handling complex design problems, it has always been the dream of plant engineers to be able to come up with an algorithm which would eventually assemble the advantages of the above cited approaches while rejecting their drawbacks. Long range predictive control algorithms (LRPC) seem to some extent to satisfy such hopes. The principle of this approach will be made clearer in the next sections.

Suffice to say here that the late 1970s witnessed the development of a number of computer control algorithms which used long-range predictions of the process output. Early work involved the development of the model algorithmic control algorithm (MAC) (Richalet *et al.*, 1978), in which the output of a linear time-invariant system at discrete time instants is described by means of a discrete impulse response. The algorithm then makes use of an approximation of this system's impulse response by a finite number of terms, which reflects the so-called *prediction horizon*.

Also during that period, the dynamic matrix control algorithm (DMC) (Cutler and Ramaker, 1980) enjoyed great popularity. Evolving from a technique that represents process dynamics with a set of numerical coefficients together with a least-squares formulation, it promised to solve complex control problems, especially those associated with systems exhibiting large dead-times.

In contrast to the MAC and DMC approaches where the process is described by dynamic impulses or step responses, the extended prediction self-adaptive control algorithm (EPSAC) (De Keyser and Van Cauwenberghe, 1979a, 1979b, 1985) uses an autoregressive moving average (ARMA) model representation of the process dynamics. The one-step ahead predictor is computed by means of a prediction model whose parameters are estimated using a recursive (extended) least-squares (RLS) method. The algorithm is also able to predict the process over a range which is usually taken greater than the maximum anticipated value of time delay. The key assumption that all future control increments are taken to be zero is one characteristic of this algorithm.

The extended adaptive control algorithm (EHAC) (Ydstie, 1984) uses almost the same parametric process model as the EPSAC version. Its fundamental idea is to compute at each sampling instant a sequence of inputs that satisfy a criterion over the chosen prediction horizon which is the only design parameter in the method.

Reported applications within industry showed that Richalet's algorithm (MAC) is unsuitable for non-minimum-phase plants, but the DMC, EPSAC and EHAC algorithms seem to be very effective. However, one criticism that was acknowledged is that they, in fact, either have a unique or relatively few design parameters. For instance, the EPSAC approach uses the prediction horizon, a weighting sequence and a model reference polynomial to accomplish a full design study, while the EHAC algorithm requires only the choice of the prediction horizon parameter. Consequently, albeit simple to formulate, the above methods do suffer from a certain loss of design flexibility vital for robustness. More recent research has seen the development of an algorithm based on the same idea of long range predictive control (LRPC) but tailored, first to retain advantages of the previously formulated algorithms, that is easy to commission, and second to add more flexibility in its design, thus leaving the user with a wider variety of parameters to arrive at the preset goal. It is known as the generalised predictive control algorithm (GPC) (Clarke *et al.*, 1987a, 1987b) and has emerged as the most popular algorithm because of several factors:

1. The model upon which it is based, which is the so-called Controlled-Autoregressive Integrated Moving Average (CARIMA) model, is effective in encountering the offset problem.

2. Its ability to predict the process behaviour over a horizon that spans that of its time delay.

3. Its inclusion of a control objective (cost function) which takes into account future errors and the weighted control effort, which is recognised to be the objective that leads to a minimum variance with a reasonable control activity.

4. Its flexibility by offering the commissioner so much latitude in reaching a fine tuning tailored to a particular application.

5. Its ability to include filtering simultaneously in control and estimation, a feature which was not possible with earlier versions of pole-placement approaches for instance.

In fact, most of these features which shape the strength of the GPC make it able to operate safely over a wide spectrum of processes which include non-minimum-phase and unstable systems, as well as those systems that include large and varying time delays, offsets, and unmodelled dynamics. Moreover, GPC's cost function allows the strategy to be extended to include the constraints imposed by the system it tries to control. Also, and unique to LRPC approaches and in particular GPC, it is possible to consider set-point predictions which can prove crucial in several areas of engineering such as robotics and biomedicine where set-point moves can be known in advance.

The widespread dissatisfaction with quantitative control among the control community seemed at one time to lure back interest to qualitative control, but advances made in model-based predictive control seem to have halted such an exodus or at least postponed it, and this is thanks to the pace set by GPC in the late 1980s, and which continues today. Several books have already been produced on this subject, the first of which is by Bitmead, Gevers and Wertz (1990) which tried to draw a comparison with the LQ approach. Others include Clarke (1994), Soeterboek (1992), and Sanchez (1995). Hence, with such an established reputation, there is no doubt that GPC's nickname of 'the universal controller' is rightfully earned, and this is the background which forms the core of the present volume which is organised into twelve related chapters, as shown in Figure 1.4, and which are outlined as follows:

- *Chapter 2.* This chapter describes the development and evaluation of SISO generalised predictive control for on-line administration of muscle relaxant drugs in operating theatres. The study considers ten patients who received surgery requiring muscle relaxation. The control system comprising the necessary hardware and software is explained and the results obtained using the GPC control strategy are presented, analysed and discussed.

- *Chapter 3.* The performance of protocols currently used for controlling the infusion of propofol, an intravenous anaesthetic, and which assumes a model based on an average pharmacokinetics population to predict the plasma concentration, is shown to degrade when mismatch conditions between the patient and the model are considered. The pharmacokinetic model is extended to include pharmacodynamics by considering mean arterial pressure measurements. Using this new extended model, the study included in this chapter assesses the performance of two control strategies, the Alvis algorithm and GPC, and draws conclusions with respect to robustness to patient parameters' mismatch, noise and disturbances.

- *Chapter 4.* Continuing with performances of GPC in the operating theatre, this chapter reviews the extension of the SISO GPC algorithm to its multivariable version by considering simultaneous adaptive control of muscle relaxation using

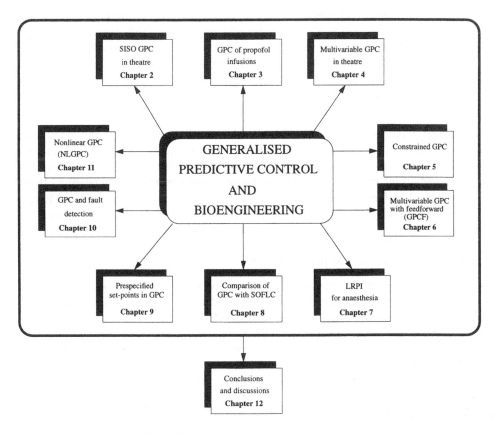

Figure 1.4   Schematic outline of the book.

the drug atracurium, together with unconsciousness via blood pressure measurements using the inhalational drug isoflurane through a number of clinical trials conducted in collaboration with Glasgow Western Infirmary. The robustness of the algorithm is evaluated through the obtained results which are thoroughly discussed.

- *Chapter 5.* The standard GPC algorithm giving the best unconstrained control sequence is found, as seen in the previous chapters, by minimising a cost function which includes the output errors as well as the control effort. While it was possible to obtain good performances with the algorithm when the input signal did not violate the maximum and minimum limits imposed by the system, parameter settings such as $NU > 1$ were found to cause the control signal to be highly active suggesting a control solution which was suboptimal. In this chapter the possibility of including such system constraints directly within the cost function to be minimised is considered by exploring the quadratic programming (QP) approach which is a powerful technique in optimisation with established convergence and stability properties. The resultant extended GPC version is presented and its performance assessed on the above multivariable anaesthesia model.

- *Chapter 6.* The issue of interactions has always represented a major challenge when it comes to designing a multivariable controller. In adaptive control, among the well-known solutions to counteract this interaction problem, the use of a P-canonical structure of the discrete model has been suggested. In this chapter another approach is proposed in which the multivariable anaesthesia model (two-input two-output) is seen as two single independent loops with the cross coupling modelled as external disturbances. The robustness of the new approach is shown via a series of simulations using the above multivariable model.

- *Chapter 7*. Adaptive controllers in general and GPC in particular rely on a good process model to achieve a good control performance by means of a recursive estimation algorithm, usually RLS. The chapter however focuses on the idea that the predictions used by the GPC controller should be made equivalent to those used by the identification strategy, in this case the strategy called Long Range Predictive Identification (LRPI). Originally formulated for SISO systems, it is extended here to the above multivariable model and in conjunction with the GPCF algorithm already presented in Chapter 6 and multivariable GPC using a P-canonical form for the process model.

- *Chapter 8*. In order to provide a comparison between modern quantitative and qualitative advanced control strategies, this chapter describes studies using GPC and Self-Organising Fuzzy Logic Control (SOFLC) on the anaesthetic multivariable model. The studies include an investigation into the ability of both algorithms to be self adapting: a key element in an intelligent system. Both paradigms are reviewed in terms of performance indices, and conclusions are drawn with respect to the algorithms' relative robustness.

- *Chapter 9*. One of the main attractive features of GPC is that it allows for changes in the set-point profile to be communicated to the algorithm some samples ahead. This interesting asset, unique to those algorithms belonging to the category of LRPC, has already proved very effective in robotics where future arm trajectories are usually known. Similarly, during surgical operations in theatre the anaesthetist, who is normally aware of the surgeon's future manipulations, can initiate the patient's muscle relaxation and depth of unconsciousness some time ahead of the surgeon's demands. This is the main thrust behind this chapter which reports on two studies. The first study deals with the SISO version of GPC to control muscle relaxation using two different patterns of set-points for typical operations which were provided by an experienced anaesthetist. The second study concerns the extension to the multivariable case involving muscle relaxation and unconsciousness. The algorithm's performance is assessed and conclusions are drawn.

- *Chapter 10*. This chapter is devoted to the merger of adaptation and intelligence. While the main thrust is an investigation of a generic architecture, the area of anaesthesia represents an ideal environment for testing the robustness of such systems in complex and nonlinear environments. The study concentrates on the following objectives:

  1. Investigating hierarchical control structures which would add intelligent supervisory layers above the basic GPC operational level.
  2. Using the above structures, incorporating the concepts of intelligent alarms for the purpose of fault diagnosis. This would include alarm conditions

covering the patient, the medical instrumentation and the computing environment.

Again, the multivariable anaesthesia model provided the main test-bed for the evaluation of such strategies.

- *Chapter 11.* All the preceding chapters describe control designs which are based on linear models using the autoregressive formulation. Current focus on MBPC research seems to be on extending the above linear formulations to nonlinear systems by including nonlinear predictions directly into the objective function. This is very much the theme of this chapter which proposes an elegant method, called Nonlinear Generalised Predictive Control (NLGPC), in which the muscle relaxant process nonlinearities which are normally embedded in a Wiener-type structure are mathematically reformulated to be taken into account in the optimisation problem. The overall algorithm is analysed and evaluated in a series of simulation experiments.

- *Chapter 12.* This chapter concludes the book by identifying the key contributions of this work, stressing the various important issues dealt with in each chapter which have been or need to be addressed, and finally by describing some current work aimed at giving a new impetus to research in the area of model-based predictive control, which also forms part of the future research directions in this area which has seen rapid and significant changes.

CHAPTER TWO

SISO Generalised Predictive Control (GPC) in Muscle Relaxation Therapy

2.1 Introduction

The major roles which are the concern of a clinical anaesthetist are those of drug-induced unconsciousness, muscle relaxation, and analgesia (i.e. pain relief). The first two roles are concentrated in the operating theatre, whereas the third role is mainly concerned with post-operative conditions. Each of these roles has been researched in recent years for the possibility of automated drug infusion via feedback strategies.

The question of measurement is a primary matter in each of the three areas of anaesthesia. The measurement of pain is the hardest of all, since it is heavily subjective, and liable to many levels of personal interpretation. However, some work has been done in this field with attempts to estimate wound healing and its associated pain level, using Kalman filtering (Jacobs *et al.*, 1982). Analgesia, when not linked to unconsciousness, will not be considered further in this chapter, since we are concerned with control principles being applied within the operating theatre. Depth of anaesthesia (i.e. unconsciousness) is hard to define, and hence to measure accurately. In practice, the anaesthetist has a number of clinical signs and on-line measurements which can be used selectively for the determination of the patient's state. Not surprisingly, therefore, a variety of methods have been used for feedback control of anaesthetic depth, based on different clinical measurements. One approach is that sensor data-fusion is required together with an on-line expert system adviser which can reason with complex, uncertain data (Linkens *et al.*, 1990).

The measurement of muscle relaxation (or drug-induced paralysis) is considerably easier. A common approach is the monitoring of evoked EMG signals produced at the hand via stimulation above the wrist. Supramaximal electrical pulse stimulation is applied, typically every 20 seconds. This stimulation ensures that all the nerve fibres are recruited, while suitable processing of the resultant EMG provides an analogue signal inversely proportional to the level of relaxation. The signal conditioning usually entails gating, rectifying and integrating. Commercial instruments are now available employing this principle, and this is the measurement basis for the work described in this chapter. An example of a typical EMG tracing is shown in Figure 2.1, which also illustrates the difficulty of good regulation when using manual control. In this example an anaesthetist attempted to control relaxation by observing the EMG signal on-line and making manual adjustments to the infusion rate. This result has also been used to elicit a human operator rule-base in fuzzy logic control of anaesthesia (Linkens and Mahfouf, 1988).

Early work on feedback control of drug infusion for muscle relaxation was performed on sheep (Cass et al., 1976). The feedback controller was based on a PID algorithm, as was the first set of human clinical trials performed by Brown et al. (1980). Similar simple control strategies have been used in more recent work using other drugs and in more extended clinical trials. Thus, Ebert et al. (1986) used a PD algorithm for vecuronium administration, and MacLeod et al. (1989) used a PI strategy for atracurium. Another emphasis has been on compact instruments for feedback control, examples being the work by Webster and Cohen (1987), and Jannett and De Falque (1990). Extreme simplification is provided by Wait et al. (1987) who merely added a relay to the output of a Datex Relaxograph alarm indicator. In this work there appeared to be no attempt to smooth the measurements or add compensation to the relay control, and obviously oscillations were continuously induced via this technique. They claimed that the levels of oscillation were surgically acceptable. To achieve this, 50% more drug consumption was indicated than in the classical PI approach used by MacLeod et al. (1989). Similar reductions in drug consumption have been indicated in simulations undertaken to compare well-regulated control schemes with the multiple bolus (this is a large drug dosage initially given by anaesthetic to patients to obtain a high level of relaxation in a relatively short time) regime calculated via the manufacturers' recommendations (Abbod, private communication). One problem with feedback control in biomedicine is that there are enormous patient-to-patient variations in dynamic model parameters. This is compounded by large time varying parameters for an individual patient during the course of an operation. This makes it difficult to design a fixed-parameter PID controller which will be suitable in all cases. This was also noted in studies on hypertension control using sodium nitroprusside by Sheppard and co-workers (Sheppard et al., 1979). Thus, in certain cases oscillations occurred, and this has also been observed in the muscle relaxation studies. This has led to the need to investigate self-adaptive control strategies, and later self-organising controllers.

To facilitate the design of advanced controllers, it is necessary to have a good mathematical model of the process. Identification studies on animals have produced model structures and parameters which confirm the wide variability and also the nonlinearity in the so-called pharmacodynamics for relaxant drugs behaviour (Linkens et al., 1982, 1985). This validated model has been used extensively in designing and simulating controllers based on either quantitative (e.g. self-tuning) or qualitative (e.g. self-organising) techniques.

An early attempt at adaptive control used a pole-placement self-tuning algorithm in animal studies (Linkens et al., 1985). In this work two non-depolarising drugs were used, and the incorporation of a Smith Predictor to offset the time delay inherent in the drug circulation was also investigated. The simple and well-known nature of the PID controller suggests that self-tuning might be applied to that structure. Although this is possible in industry, the normal method of iterative adjustment of parameters via deliberately induced oscillations or large disturbances is not acceptable in operating theatre. An alternative model-based self-tuning PID approach has

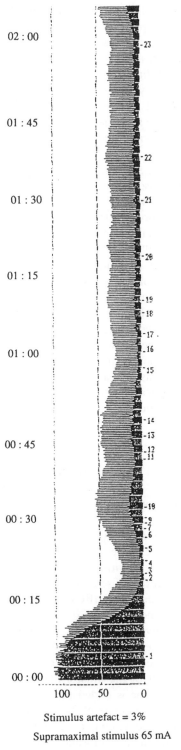

Stimulus artefact = 3%

Supramaximal stimulus 65 mA

Figure 2.1 Typical Relaxograph EMG tracing obtained during manual control of drug infusion. The light bars indicate the level of relaxation.

been developed and evaluated clinically by Denai *et al.* (1990). This particular strategy is limited to systems with pure time delay and second-order dynamics, and is relevant for muscle relaxant control. Another model-based approach due to Olkkola and Schwilden (1991) used an average population pharmacokinetic model, which was updated periodically on-line and then used for predictive control of drug administration. Earlier work by Rametti and co-workers had considered a dual-mode controller, with different strategies being adopted for initial and regulation phases for relaxation control. The initial phase controller used a sequence of small bolus doses, the amounts being adjusted to minimise the risk of excessive overshoot in the paralysis level (Rametti, 1985; Rametti *et al.*, 1985). This protocol is not normally acceptable in theatre, and later work (Bradlow and O'Mahony, 1990) has emphasised the regulation phase controller which comprises a state and parameter estimator which is used predictively to calculate the best current dosage.

Common to much of the above work is the theme of predictive control, and this is the background to the present chapter which investigates generalised predictive control (GPC) (Clarke *et al.*, 1987a, 1987b) for on-line muscle relaxant drug administration. GPC has advantages over other forms of self-tuning control in that it is robust against variable and unknown time delay, overparameterisation of system models, and has good disturbance rejection properties. It does, however, have a number of design 'knobs' which must be adjusted carefully to suit the particular application. In the following sections a mathematical model for the pharmacology of atracurium is developed, together with off-line simulations of GPC based on this model. Design values were then transferred to an on-line simulation running 60 times faster than real time. This validated software and hardware system was then transferred to the operating theatre, and the resulting clinical trials and their evaluation are described in later sections.

2.2 Physiological background pertaining to the muscle relaxation process

2.2.1 Neuromuscular transmission

In the chain of events that starts with the stimulation of a motor nerve and ends with the contraction of a muscle, the most crucial link is the synapse between the nerve and the muscle – the neuromuscular junction. As shown in Figure 2.2, the motor nerve is separated from the muscle by the synaptic cleft. This cleft is, in fact, a sub-division of the extracellular fluid (ECF) from which it is separated by the Schwann cell membrane. The neurotransmitter acetylcholine (Ach) is responsible for transmitting motor nerve activity across this junction. Early work by Birks *et al.* (1960) elucidated the fundamental anatomy of the neuromuscular junction, and modern techniques have allowed refinements of details relative to this structure. The motor nerve ends at that part of the muscle membrane known as the motor end plate. In this area, the membrane is folded into longitudinal gutters; the ridges of each gutter conceal orifices to secondary clefts. Around these orifices, a high concentration of a chemical substance known as acetylcholinesterase (AchE) has been proved to be present. The end plate membrane potential is a reflection of the uneven distribution of ions across the surface membrane. In its resting state, this membrane is far more permeable to potassium ions (K^+) than those of sodium (Na^+) (ratio of

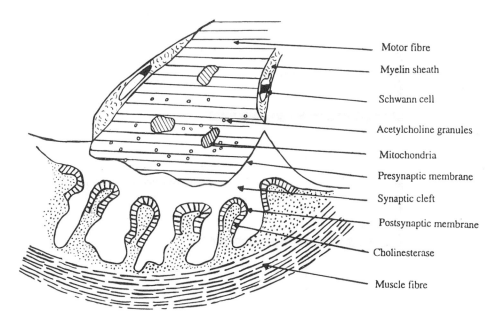

Motor fibre

Myelin sheath

Schwann cell

Acetylcholine granules

Mitochondria

Presynaptic membrane

Synaptic cleft

Postsynaptic membrane

Cholinesterase

Muscle fibre

Figure 2.2 Schematic representation of the neuromuscular junction.

100). As a result, (K^+) ions pass out of the cell along their concentration gradient until the accumulation of positively charged ions on the outside of the membrane causes an opposing force to further migrations of potassium ions (K^+). The inside of the membrane has a negative potential, whereas the outside has a positive electrical charge. The membrane is said to be polarised. The transmembrane potential reaches a value of -70 mV to -90 mV. The arrival of an impulse at the nerve terminals causes the release of the chemical substance Ach (Dale and Feldberg, 1934) which causes the opening of the sodium pores by reacting with specialised receptors on the post-synaptic membrane. This causes depolarisation of the post-synaptic membrane by increasing its permeability to (Na^+) ions relative to (K^+) ions. The end plate potential is reversed giving rise to an action potential propagation and subsequent muscle contraction. These events are quickly terminated as a result of interactions between Ach and AchE present in the orifices of the secondary clefts.

2.2.2 Muscle relaxant drugs and their mechanism of action

As seen in the previous section, the synaptic gap is the site which witnesses the activity leading to a muscle contraction. Therefore, the process of neuromuscular transmission can only be blocked if relaxant drugs gain access to the synaptic cleft and break the previously described chain of events which are summarised in Figure 2.3. Depending on their mechanism of action, muscle relaxant agents fall into two categories: depolarising and non-depolarising drugs. Depolarising drugs such as suxamethonium and decamethonium are believed to act by producing a continuous depolarisation of the post-synaptic membrane, rendering it unresponsive to Ach and at their first application a voluntary muscle contracts, but unlike Ach, these agents

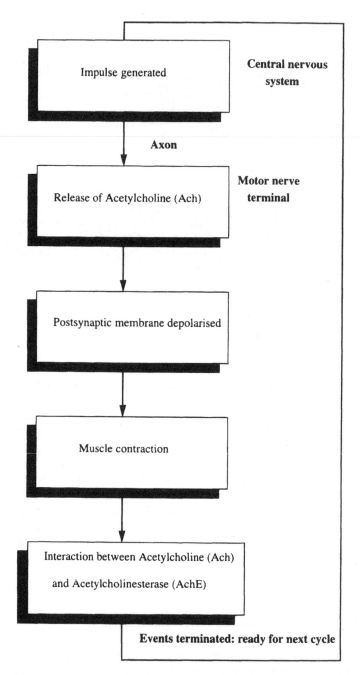

Figure 2.3   Schematic diagram showing the chain of events leading to muscle relaxation.

are not destroyed by cholinesterase and the depolarisation is maintained. Non-depolarising agents, however, compete with Ach for the cholinoreceptors. As a result, when Ach reacts with these drugs, it fails to cause sufficient sodium pores to open to allow threshold depolarisation to take place. These agents do not induce muscle pain following their administration and because of this they are preferred to the other category. Atracurium, a non-depolarising fast acting agent which has gained popularity over pancuronium and d-tubocurarine, is the subject of this research study and its associated mathematical model is presented next.

2.3   Atracurium mathematical model

In order to identify the muscle relaxation process associated with drugs, pharmacological modelling is commonly used to describe the metabolism of such drugs. Pharmacological modelling comprises two main categories known as pharmacokinetics and pharmacodynamics. Pharmacokinetics studies the relationship that exists between drug dose and drug concentration in the blood plasma as well as other parts of the body. Interpretation of this relationship can be given a mathematical meaning via the concept of compartmental models. Using this concept the body consists of several compartments each representing one part of the body that involves the drug metabolism. Pharmacodynamics, however, is concerned with the drug concentration in the blood and the effect produced. One key postulate of this is that there is a considerable delay separating the first administration of a muscle relaxant drug and the onset of relaxation; this nonlinear effect is known as the 'margin of safety' (Paton and Waud, 1967; Waud and Waud, 1971), whereby no depression of twitch response can be detected until over 75% of the receptors are occluded. Also, because of saturation effects, once initiated, paralysis cannot increase indefinitely as the drug dosage increases.

2.3.1   Pharmacokinetics

It has been shown that after a drug injection, the plasma concentration of atracurium declines rapidly in two exponential phases corresponding to distribution and elimination (Ward *et al.*, 1983). Therefore, a conventional two-compartment model is used by adding an elimination path from the peripheral compartment obeying the so-called Hofmann elimination (Ward *et al.*, 1983; Weatherly *et al.*, 1983). Figure 2.4 is a schematic diagram showing the different model components.

If x_i is the drug concentration at time t, $\dot{x}_i$ its rate of change, and u the drug input, then:

$$\dot{x}_1 = -(k_{10} + k_{12})x_1 + k_{21}x_2 + u$$
$$\dot{x}_2 = k_{12}x_1 - (k_{20} + k_{21})x_2 \tag{2.1}$$

Using Laplace transforms, equation (2.1) can be rewritten as:

$$sX_1 = -(k_{10} + k_{12})X_1 + k_{21}X_2 + U$$
$$sX_2 = k_{12}X_1 - (k_{20} + k_{21})X_2 \tag{2.2}$$

Hence,

$$\frac{X_1(s)}{U(s)} = \frac{s + k_{20} + k_{21}}{(s + k_{10} + k_{12})(s + k_{20} + k_{21}) - k_{12}k_{21}} \tag{2.3}$$

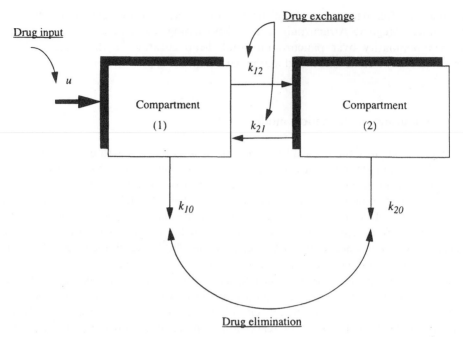

Figure 2.4   A two-compartment model for atracurium with an additional elimination path (k_{20}).

Experimental studies by Weatherley *et al.* (1983) gave the following mean values for the pharmacokinetic parameters:

$$k_{12} + k_{10} = 0.26 \text{ min}^{-1}$$

$$k_{21} + k_{20} = 0.094 \text{ min}^{-1}$$

$$k_{12} \times k_{21} = 0.015 \text{ min}^{-2}$$

Substituting in equation (2.3) leads to:

$$\frac{X_1(s)}{U(s)} = \frac{9.94(1 + 10.64s)}{(1 + 3.08s)(1 + 34.42s)} \tag{2.4}$$

which describes the pharmacokinetics of the muscle relaxation system relating to the drug atracurium in a transfer function form.

2.3.2 Pharmacodynamics

Simultaneous identification of pharmacokinetics and pharmacodynamics of d-tubo-curarine (Sheiner *et al.*, 1979) led to the findings that the dynamics of the drug effect do not coincide with those of the plasma concentration. Similarly, in order to characterise temporal aspects of drug effect, a third compartment known as the 'effect compartment' has been introduced. It is connected to the central compartment by a first-order rate constant k_{1E}, whereas the rate constant k_{E0} characterises the drug dissipation from the effect compartment, as shown in Figure 2.5.

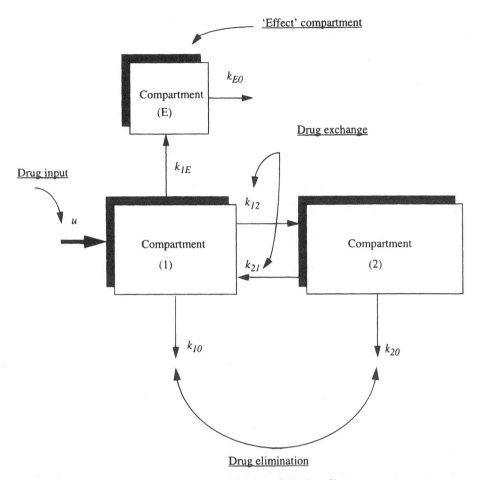

Figure 2.5 Modification of the atracurium kinetics to include the 'effect' compartment E.

In this latter compartment, the drug concentration change is governed by the following equation:

$$\dot{x}_E = k_{1E} x_1 - k_{E0} x_E \tag{2.5}$$

Using Laplace transforms yields:

$$X_E = \frac{k_{1E} X_1}{s + k_{E0}} \tag{2.6}$$

The Hill equation (Weatherley *et al.*, 1983; Whiting and Kelman, 1980) may be used to relate the effect to a specific blood concentration of drug:

$$E_{\text{eff}} = \frac{E_{\text{max}}}{1 + \dfrac{X_E(50)^\alpha}{X_E^\alpha}} \tag{2.7}$$

where X_E is the drug concentration and $X_E(50)$ is the drug concentration at a 50% effect.

Experimental work (Whiting and Kelman, 1980; Weatherley *et al.*, 1983) has given the following parameters:

$$k_{E0} = 0.208 \text{ min}^{-1}$$

$$X_E(50) = 0.404 \text{ } \mu g \text{ ml}^{-1}$$

$$\alpha = 2.98$$

$$k_{1E} = 10^{-4} \text{ min}^{-1}$$

Combining equations (2.6) and (2.4) and normalising the overall open-loop gain at 1.0 leads to:

$$\frac{X_E}{U} = \frac{K(1 + T_4 s) \text{ e}^{-\tau s}}{(1 + T_1 s)(1 + T_2 s)(1 + T_3 s)} \tag{2.8}$$

where $K = 1$; $\tau = 1$ min; $T_1 = 4.81$ min; $T_2 = 34.42$ min; $T_3 = 3.08$ min; $T_4 = 10.64$ min.

Finally, the overall nonlinear model is obtained by combining equation (2.8) together with the Hill equation (2.7), or alternatively a dead-space in series with a saturation element.

2.4 Development of the adaptive GPC algorithm

Long range prediction algorithms enjoyed considerable popularity in the late 1970s especially with the development of a computer control algorithm called dynamic matrix control (DMC) (Cutler and Ramaker, 1980). Evolving from a technique that represents process dynamics with a set of numerical coefficients together with a least-squares formulation, it promised to solve complex control problems, especially those associated with systems exhibiting large dead-times. DMC's use of a non-parametric model was later challenged by another multi-step long range predictive control algorithm: generalised predictive control (GPC) (Clarke *et al.*, 1987a, 1987b). It is a natural successor to the generalised minimum variance (GMV) design (Clarke and Gawthrop, 1975), and is considered to be very robust. Its development is reviewed in the next section.

2.4.1 Model description

The so-called CARMA (Controlled Autoregressive Moving Average) model (Wellstead, 1980; Clarke and Gawthrop, 1975) has found its place in many self-tuning designs, whereby an integrator is inserted in an ad hoc fashion to counteract any offset that may occur when regulating a process around a non-zero set-point. Another method suggested the use of a CARIMA (controlled autoregressive integrated moving average) model (Belanger, 1983; Tuffs and Clarke, 1985), in which the noise term is non-stationary. Good adaptive behaviour has been shown to be possible for this case.

Consider the following locally linearised discrete model in the backward shift operator z^{-1}:

$$A(z^{-1})y(t) = B(z^{-1})u(t - 1) + x(t) \tag{2.9}$$

where

$$A(z^{-1}) = 1 + a_1 z^{-1} + a_2 z^{-2} + \ldots + a_n z^{-n}$$
$$B(z^{-1}) = z^{-k}(b_1 + b_2 z^{-1} + b_3 z^{-2} + \ldots + b_m z^{-m+1})$$

and z^{-1} represents the backward shift operator; $u(t)$ the control input; $y(t)$ the measured variable; k the assumed value of time delay. $x(t)$ represents the disturbance upon which the model is based and is considered to be of moving average form, i.e.:

$$x(t) = C(z^{-1}) \frac{\xi(t)}{\Delta} \tag{2.10}$$

where

$$C(z^{-1}) = c_0 + c_1 z^{-1} + c_2 z^{-2} + \ldots + c_p z^{-p}$$

$\xi(t) =$ an uncorrelated random sequence

$\Delta = 1 - z^{-1}$

Thus, substituting equation (2.10) into equation (2.9) and appending the operator Δ gives:

$$A(z^{-1})\Delta y(t) = B(z^{-1})\Delta u(t-1) + C(z^{-1})\xi(t) \tag{2.11}$$

2.4.2 The control law

Before describing the mathematical background behind the algorithm, it is worthwhile outlining briefly the theory of long range predictive control.

The strategy illustrated in Figure 2.6 can be summarised as follows (De Keyser and Van Cauwenberghe, 1983):

- At each present time t a forecast is made of the process output over a long-range time horizon by means of a mathematical model of the process dynamics.
- Several control actions will be proposed as a result of this forecast, but only the best strategy will be selected according to the predefined set-point.
- The chosen candidate is then applied as the control action at the same time t. The whole procedure is again repeated at the next sample. This procedure is also known as the 'receding horizon approach'.

The controller therefore computes the vector of controls using optimisation of a function of the form:

$$\begin{cases} J = E[(Q1 + Q2)] \\ Q1 = \sum_{j=N_1}^{N_2} [(P(z^{-1})\hat{y}(t+j) - \omega(t+j))^2] \\ Q2 = \sum_{j=1}^{NU} [\lambda(j)(\Delta u(t+j-1))^2] \end{cases} \tag{2.12}$$

where N_1 is the minimum costing horizon; N_2 is the maximum costing horizon; NU is the control horizon; ω is the future set-points usually presumed known; and $\lambda(j)$ is the control weighting sequence.

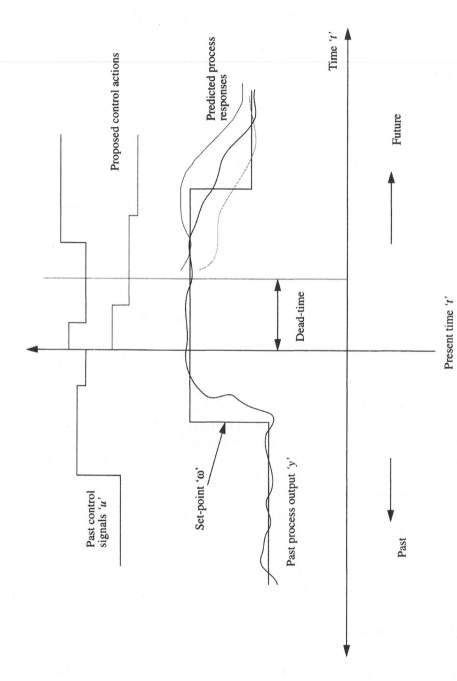

Figure 2.6 Long range predictive control (LRPC) principle.

Omitting z^{-1} for the sake of brevity, one can write:

$$P\hat{y}(t+j) = \bar{\bar{G}}_j \Delta u(t+j-1) + \Psi(t+j) \tag{2.13}$$

$$\Psi(t+j) = \bar{G}_j \Delta u^f(t-1) - \bar{F}_j y^f(t) \tag{2.14}$$

$$TP = E_j A\Delta + z^{-j}\bar{F}_j \tag{2.15}$$

$$P(z^{-1}) = \frac{P_n(z^{-1})}{P_d(z^{-1})} \quad (P(1)=1) \tag{2.16}$$

$$T(z^{-1}) = 1 + t_1 z^{-1} + \ldots + t_{nt} z^{-nt} \tag{2.17}$$

$$\bar{F}_j = \frac{F_j}{P_d} \tag{2.18}$$

$$E_j B = \bar{\bar{G}}_j T + z^{-j}\bar{G}_j \tag{2.19}$$

$$\bar{\bar{G}}_j = \bar{\bar{g}}_0 + \bar{\bar{g}}_1 z^{-1} + \ldots + \bar{\bar{g}}_{j-1} z^{-j+1}$$

$$\bar{G}_j = \bar{g}_{j0} + \bar{g}_{j1} z^{-1} + \ldots + \bar{g}_{j(i-1)} z^{-i+1}$$

$$i = \text{from 1 to } \max(\delta B, \delta T)$$

$$1 \le j \le N_2$$

where subscript f denotes signals filtered by $1/T(z^{-1})$.

P and T are user-chosen polynomials in z^{-1}. $1/T(z^{-1})$ is chosen as a low-pass filter, and is the so-called observer polynomial for the predictor of equation (2.14) (Astrom and Wittenmark, 1984). P is referred to as the model-following polynomial and the condition $P(1) = 1$ ensures an offset-free response (Clarke, 1985).

The minimisation of the cost function described in equation (2.12) leads to the following projected control increment:

$$\Delta u(t) = \bar{g}^T(\omega - \Psi) \tag{2.20}$$

where $\Psi = [\Psi(t+N_1), \ldots, \Psi(t+N_2)]$, $\bar{g}^T$ is the first row of the matrix $(G_d^T G_d + \lambda I)^{-1} G_d^T$, and G_d is the dynamic (step-response) matrix of the form given in Clarke et al. (1987a).

2.5 Simulation studies

The simulation studies have been undertaken in two parts, the first being concerned with implementation of the GPC algorithm on a SUN workstation. The second consisted of evaluating the algorithm under real time conditions using a VIDAC 336 analog computer.

2.5.1 Implementation of the GPC algorithm on a SUN workstation

The overall nonlinear muscle relaxant model describing atracurium dynamics was simulated, such that for the continuous model being considered, a fourth-order Runge–Kutta method with fixed step length was used for the numerical integration together with a sampling period of 1 minute. The pharmacokinetics of the drug are given by the three-time constant transfer function with a unit time delay of equation

(2.8), whereas the pharmacodynamics are modelled by the Hill equation (2.7). Whenever the controller is operating in the nonlinear region, parameter estimation is frozen and control is maintained with a fixed PI controller, and the self-tuner takes over as soon as the nonlinear region is traversed. Figure 2.7 illustrates the structure of the overall control strategy.

As pointed out earlier, because the system exhibits a large dead-zone, a fixed PI controller, which includes gains obtained via optimisation using a program called PSI (van den Bosch, 1979), provides initial control for 20 sampling periods after which the self-adaptive GPC took over. Parameter estimation, using incremental data, takes the form of a UD-factorisation algorithm (Bierman, 1977) which is a modified robust version of the well-known RLS algorithm. A third-order discrete-time model was estimated with an assumed time delay of 1 minute, i.e.:

$$G_1(z^{-1}) = z^{-1} \frac{b_1 z^{-1} + b_2 z^{-2} + b_3 z^{-3}}{1 + a_1 z^{-1} + a_2 z^{-2} + a_3 z^{-3}} \tag{2.21}$$

Parameter estimates were all set to 0.0 unless otherwise specified, the covariance matrix was made equal to $Cov = 10^4 . I$ and a value of $\rho = 0.95$ was adopted for the forgetting factor. The control signal was clipped between maximum and minimum values of respectively 0.0 and 1.0. These limitations were also reflected back to the estimator by recomputing the actual control sequence which was asserted (Clarke, 1985).

The experiments were conducted in two phases. Phase 1 utilised the basic GPC algorithm (Clarke *et al.*, 1987a), while phase 2 was concerned with the extended algorithm (Clarke *et al.*, 1987b) using the observer polynomial $T(z^{-1})$.

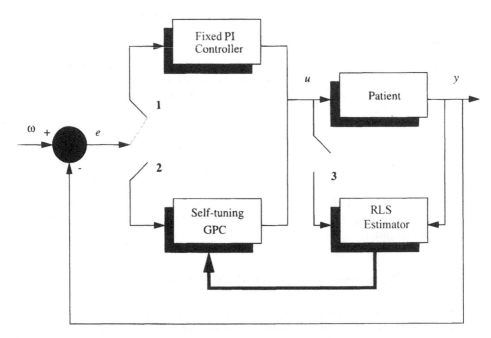

Figure 2.7 Schematic diagram representing the overall structure of the muscle relaxation control system; switch 1: on for 20 minutes; switch 2: on after 20 minutes; switch 3: on when output greater than 0.10 and less than 0.95.

The performance of the self-adaptive GPC algorithm under the above initial and jacketing conditions together with a combination of (1, 10, 1, 0) for (N_1, N_2, NU, λ) is shown in Figure 2.8. The set-point command signal was 80% then 70% every 100 samples. The parameter estimates converged to the following final values:

$$\hat{a}_1 = -2.149 \quad \hat{a}_2 = 1.511 \quad \hat{a}_3 = -0.349$$
$$\hat{b}_1 = 0.010 \quad \hat{b}_2 = 0.002 \quad \hat{b}_3 = -0.005$$

These are equivalent to the following positions in the z-plane:

zeros: -0.85; 0.62

poles: 0.92; $(0.61 \pm 0.04 \text{ i})$

These values could be considered as reflecting the compartmental idea since the imaginary part of the conjugate poles is a negligible quantity compared to the real part.

In muscle relaxation, a pure time delay has been shown to occur due to the transport of blood via the circulation system (Linkens et al., 1982). Its value has been shown experimentally to vary from subject to subject with a ratio of approximately 4:1. To simulate such a situation, an experiment was conducted in which the dead-time value τ in equation (2.8) was made to vary from 1 minute to 4 minutes every 100 samples. A noise sequence in the form of a pseudo-random binary sequence (PRBS) with 1% amplitude was superimposed on the output. The same

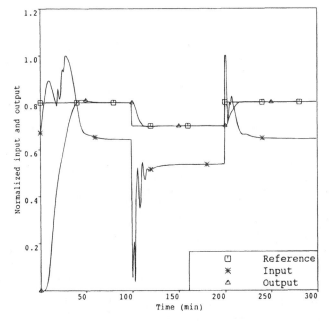

Figure 2.8 Closed-loop response to atracurium model under self-tuning GPC algorithm with $N_1 = 1$; $N_2 = 10$; $NU = 1$ (the vertical axis is scaled in such a way that an output of 0 represents no paralysis whereas an output of 1.0 represents total paralysis, in contrast to the Relaxograph tracings where 0% represents total paralysis and 100% represents no paralysis, as in Figure 2.1).

combination for the controller parameters was considered except that an observer polynomial $T(z^{-1})$ of the form $T(z^{-1}) = 1 - 0.97\ z^{-1}$, where 0.97 corresponds to the dominant time constant of the process, was included this time, and any time delay variations in the process were represented in the $B(z^{-1})$ polynomial by estimating three extra 'b' coefficients, i.e.:

$$G_1(z^{-1}) = z^{-1}\ \frac{b_1 z^{-1} + b_2 z^{-2} + b_3 z^{-3} + b_4 z^{-4} + b_5 z^{-5} + b_6 z^{-6}}{1 + a_1 z^{-1} + a_2 z^{-2} + a_3 z^{-3}} \qquad (2.22)$$

The result of the run is shown in Figure 2.9 with the algorithm maintaining good control in spite of the noise and the changing delay occurring at the same time as the changing operating point.

2.5.2   Microcomputer implementation of the GPC algorithm

To validate further the performance of the GPC algorithm, it was considered necessary to assess its capabilities under real-time conditions. In fact, previous research studies demonstrated this procedure to be very useful prior to any trials in theatre (Denai *et al.*, 1990; Menad, 1984), providing software and hardware validation for the system.

The real-time simulation study was undertaken by combining a microcomputer system and a VIDAC 336 analog computer. Interfacing between the two devices was via 10 bits ADC and DAC hardware converters. Synchronisation between the hard-

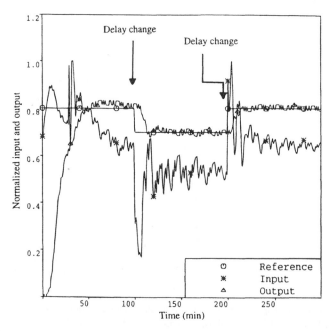

Figure 2.9   Closed-loop response of atracurium model with additive noise: extended GPC algorithm with $N_1 = 1$; $N_2 = 10$; $NU = 1$ and $T(z^{-1}) = 1 - 0.97\ z^{-1}$.

ware and software was established by the interrupt routines which set up the built-in real-time clock from the background processing unit. The frequency of the interrupts on all the channels (AD/DA) was chosen to be 1 Hz corresponding to a sampling time 60 times faster than real-time performance.

In order to keep the processing time below the time period between interrupts (less than 1 second) the estimated discrete-time model was reduced to order 2, whereas any change in the delay due to the hardware was enhanced in the $B(z^{-1})$ polynomial, i.e.:

$$G_1(z^{-1}) = \frac{b_1 z^{-1} + b_2 z^{-2} + b_3 z^{-3} + b_4 z^{-4}}{1 + a_1 z^{-1} + a_2 z^{-2}} \tag{2.23}$$

This can be done safely with the GPC structure since the algorithm allows the use of the observer polynomial $T(z^{-1})$ to compensate for any unmodelled dynamics (Clarke *et al.*, 1987b). The choice of the filter was a trade-off between good disturbance rejection properties and an acceptable overall performance (Robinson and Clarke, 1991). Thus, a first-order polynomial of the form $T(z^{-1}) = 1 - 0.8\, z^{-1}$ was adopted throughout. Due to limited space only one experiment will be described here.

The patient population can be divided into three categories of high, medium and low drug sensitivity corresponding respectively to a high, average and low gain. This gain variability, as well as variability in the dynamics, is reckoned to be due to factors affecting drug disposition into the body, or the ability of the organs of the body to respond to a particular drug concentration. The gain, particularly, can also vary for one patient on-line, and the self-adaptive GPC should not exhibit any

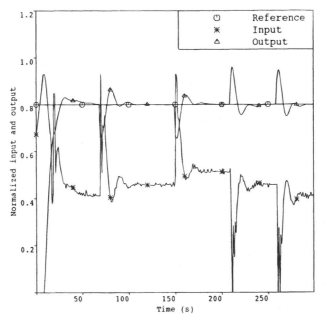

Figure 2.10a Closed-loop response of atracurium model with additive gain change disturbances at iterations 70, 150, 210 seconds.

unstable mode as a result of this. To test the robustness of the algorithm under such conditions, a run was conducted in which the open-loop gain was made to vary on-line in rapid steps from 1.00 to 0.90 at iteration 70, from 0.90 to 0.80 at iteration 150, from 0.80 to 0.90 at iteration 210, and finally back to 1.00 at iteration 260. Conditions for the estimator and jacketing were similar to those previously considered and a combination of $(1, 10, 1, 0)$ was chosen for (N_1, N_2, NU, λ). Figure 2.10a shows how the GPC, with the help of the observer polynomial $T(z^{-1})$, rejected the four disturbances quickly without deteriorating its performance despite the harsh changes. The variations of the parameter estimates illustrated in Figure 2.10b showed little drift in the dynamics, whereas the $\hat{b}$ estimates changed appropriately,

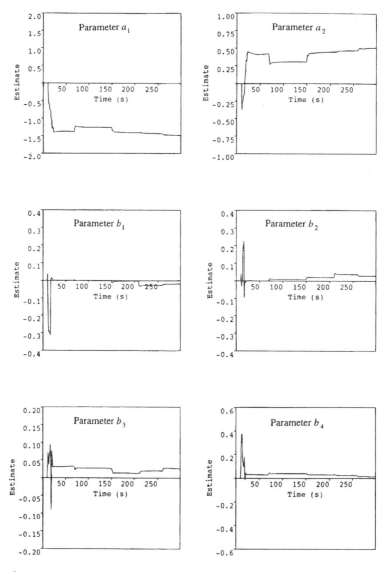

Figure 2.10b   System parameter estimates corresponding to Figure 2.10a.

Table 2.1 Model parameter estimates for an on-line varying gain

Parameter estimates convergence

Parameter estimates	Time-phase (from … to …) (s)			
	0–70	71–150	151–260	261–300
a_1	−1.3208	−1.2925	−1.4371	−1.4824
a_2	0.3613	0.3346	0.4677	0.5105
b_1	−0.0001	−0.0051	−0.0263	0.0181
b_2	0.0023	0.0126	0.0371	0.0283
b_3	0.0295	0.0236	0.0195	0.0262
b_4	0.0359	0.0394	0.0221	0.0131
Gain	**1.75**	**1.67**	**1.71**	**1.76**
TC_1	**1.05**	**0.97**	**1.43**	**1.64**
TC_2	**14.63**	**14.74**	**15.90**	**15.72**

i.e. a decrease in their value whenever the gain decreased, and an increase whenever the gain increased. Table 2.1 summarises the values of the parameter estimates at the end of each phase, as well as the gain and time constants of the corresponding continuous-time system.

The conditions under which the GPC algorithm was investigated were closely related to reality, as far as the uncertainty of the model parameters were concerned, which themselves reflect variability of patient parameters. The controller proved very robust in making the output track the set-point command efficiently despite nonlinearities, and also coping with offsets induced by the hardware. These latter conditions emphasised the realistic character of the simulations. Corresponding control signals were reasonably active, due to the observer polynomial $T(z^{-1})$ which clearly attenuated the high frequency components originating from the hardware, and later amplified by the Δ operator. Finally, it should be noted that these real-time simulations were very useful in assessing the robustness of the algorithm over a wide range of subjects' parameters (Mahfouf, 1991) before its implementation and evaluation in the operating theatre. The transfer of the controller, whose validated software remained on the microcomputer, to a clinical environment is described in the next section.

2.6 Performance of GPC in the operating theatre

The muscle relaxation control system used in the operating theatre during surgery is illustrated in Figure 2.11 and consisted of the following components:

- A microcomputer system which incorporates the control algorithm.
- A Datex Relaxograph system for measuring the degree of muscle relaxation (paralysis) by electrically stimulating a peripheral nerve and displaying the resulting EMG (electromyogram) response. Equipped with five electrodes, it employs the train-of-four principle (TOF) and features an automatic search for supramaximal stimulation current level. Stimuli of the TOF sequence are given

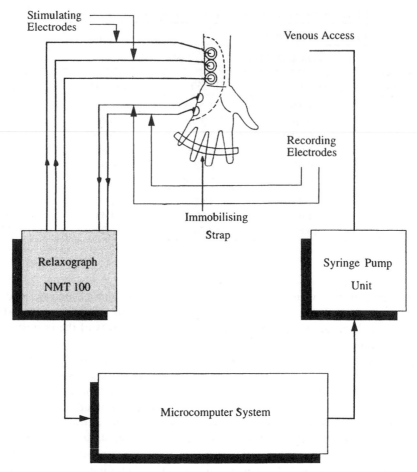

Figure 2.11   Schematic diagram representing the muscle relaxation control system used in the operating theatre.

at a rate of two pulses per second every 20 seconds. The device displays $T1\%$ and $TR\%$ values given by the following formulae:

$$T1 = \frac{\text{first twitch}}{\text{control}} \times 100\%$$

$$TR = \frac{\text{last twitch}}{\text{first twitch}} \times 100\% = \text{TOF ratio}$$

In this case $T1$ represents the value of the EMG level.

- A digital pump driving a disposable 50 ml/60 ml syringe containing a solution of atracurium.

The links between the computer, the Relaxograph device and the syringe pump drive unit were via the serial and parallel input–output ports.

2.6.1 The control algorithm and the sampling period

Because the Relaxograph delivers signals only at precise intervals of 20 seconds, a change in the existing program had to be made to facilitate the use of a 1 minute sampling interval which was found to give adequate results both in simulations and in real-time experiments. This was done by using a three-point non-recursive averaging filter of the form:

$$G_{AF}(z^{-1}) = \frac{1}{3}\sum_{i=0}^{2} z^{-i} \tag{2.24}$$

where

$$z^{-1} = e^{-sh}$$

$$h = 20 \text{ seconds} \tag{2.25}$$

The log-magnitude plot response of the filter is shown in Figure 2.12, with the characteristic having a -3 dB point at 0.008 Hz. This provides low-pass filtering which reduces signal artefacts caused by fluctuations in the response due to inadequate positioning of the stimulating and recording electrodes and diathermy (severe electrical interference).

When closed-loop control is established, a PI controller is used to provide initial control allowing the parameter estimation routine to gather sufficient identification data. The PI parameters were obtained using Ziegler–Nichols techniques (Ziegler and Nichols, 1942) applied to open-loop step responses in an off-line study. The dose of atracurium is expressed in ml h^{-1} and is obtained using the following

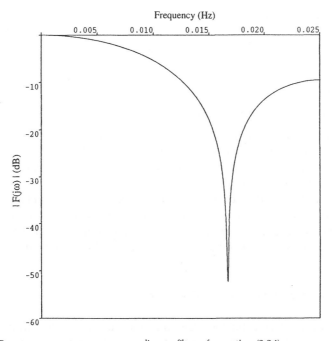

Figure 2.12 Frequency response corresponding to filter of equation (2.24).

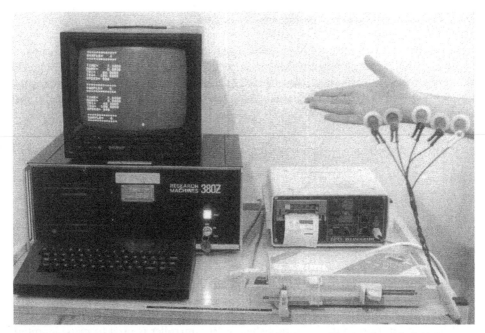

Figure 2.13   Patient in the anaesthetic room connected to the overall control system which includes (clockwise) the microcomputer system, the Datex Relaxograph, and the CRITIKON syringe pump.

formula:

$$I \text{ (ml h}^{-1}) = K_p e + K_i(\textstyle\sum e + PL) \qquad\qquad (2.26)$$

where

$$K_p = k_p W_t$$
$$K_i = k_i W_t$$
$$k_p = 0.02 \text{ kg}^{-1}, \qquad k_i = 0.0021 \text{ kg}^{-1}$$

I is the atracurium infusion rate, W_t represents the actual patient's weight, whereas e is the difference between the actual $T1\%$ and the target $T1\%$.

These values were also used as a basis for an algorithm successfully applied in theatre by Denai *et al.* (1990).

At this stage it is worth noting that when a bolus dose is preloaded to induce muscle relaxation, the PI controller is initialised with some integral value PL, so as to shorten the stabilisation period when the closed-loop control mode is entered. Nominal values between 150 and 333 were used throughout the trials for PL.

2.6.2   Clinical preparation of patients before surgery

The patients were selected on the basis that they did not suffer from any known sensitivity to anaesthetic drugs or myoneural disorders, and had not been taking drugs known to affect neuromuscular transmission. They all underwent abdominal or orthopaedic surgery which normally requires muscle relaxation.

Approximately 60 minutes before surgery, they were premedicated with temazepam by mouth. Anaesthesia was induced with methohexitane 1 mg kg^{-1}. The trachea was intubated when $T1$ reached a value between 10% and 15%. The lungs were inflated with 30% oxygen, 70% nitrous oxide and 1% enflurane. During surgery, enflurane anaesthesia was supplemented with boluses of fentanyl at 1 μg kg^{-1}. While the patient was still in the anaesthetic room, the Relaxograph electrodes were carefully placed on the patient's arm, then the calibration proceeded. Once transferred to the theatre, the patient, already connected to the control system, was intravenously given an initial bolus dose of atracurium of 0.15 to 0.25 mg kg^{-1}.

The on-line controlled infusion was started when $T1$ (induced by the initial bolus) reached a level judged adequate by the anaesthetist (usually 10% to 15% of the baseline value. A 100% EMG corresponds to a 0% paralysis, whereas 0% EMG is equivalent to maximum paralysis). The muscle relaxation level was monitored until the surgeon requested cessation of paralysis. The control was then switched off immediately, and residual blockade was reversed using antagonist agents such as neostigmine (2.5 mg) and atropine (0.8 mg). Figure 2.13 is a picture taken in hospital showing a patient connected to the overall muscle relaxation control system prior to undergoing surgery.

2.6.3 Results and discussions

After local Ethics Committee approval, ten patients (eight females, two males) were selected as being suitable for the experiments. Information relating to the patients is presented in Table 2.2. The atracurium concentrations used were all 1 mg ml^{-1} unless otherwise specified.

All ten trials were conducted using a sampling-time interval of 1 minute. Consequently, the three-point non-recursive averaging filter was included in all experiments. Control and estimation were performed at 1 minute intervals, while EMG

Table 2.2 Summary of each patient's personal details

Personal details					
Patient	Sex	Age (years)	Weight (kg)	Duration of procedure (min)	Duration of control (min)
1	F	68	50	107	67
2	F	33	60	56	30
3	F	21	68	60	45
4	F	69	50	120	69
5	F	65	58	66	33
6	F	37	60	58	32
7	F	17	56	165	130
8	M	32	69	90	52
9	M	46	73	177	106
10	F	41	71	63	22

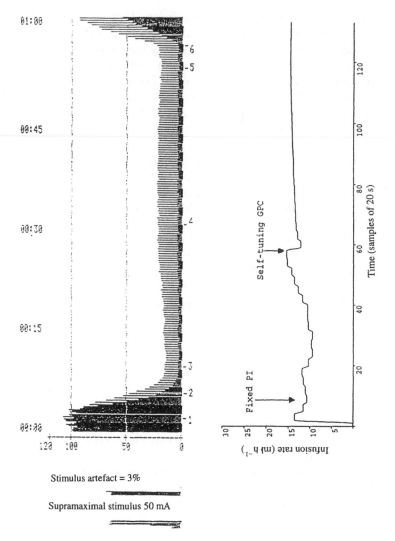

Figure 2.14a   Patient 3: recorded EMG and pump infusion rate during surgery.

readings were obtained every 20 seconds. Parameter estimation was based on the UD-factorisation algorithm and was triggered at the same time as the closed-loop control was established with a covariance matrix and forgetting factor values of $Cov = 10.I$ and $\rho = 0.999$ respectively. A 20% reference EMG level ($T1\%$) was required by the operating surgeon in all trials except for the last case corresponding to patient 10, where a 15% EMG reference level was targeted. Results corresponding to each patient are presented in two parts. The first part consists of two traces: the upper trace representing the recorded EMG level ($T1\%$), whereas the lower trace shows the variations of the infusion rate of atracurium in ml h^{-1}. The time axis is labelled in samples of 20 seconds, and it is worth noting that the infusion rate is constant over three samples of 20 seconds each. The second part of the results includes variations of the parameter estimates plotted at 1 minute intervals. Due to limited space only some of the ten experiments will be described here, illustrating the lessons learned from the trials.

Patient 3

For this experiment, whose results are shown in Figure 2.14a, the atracurium drug concentration was halved to 500 μg ml^{-1}. The controller assumed a combination of (1, 30, 1, 0) for (N_1, N_2, NU, λ) and a second-order observer polynomial $T(z^{-1}) = (1 - 0.7 z^{-1})^2$. However, the estimator assumed a third-order model with a minimum time delay of 1 minute. Mark 1 and Mark 2 on the upper trace of the same figure represent the times at which the anaesthetist administered bolus doses

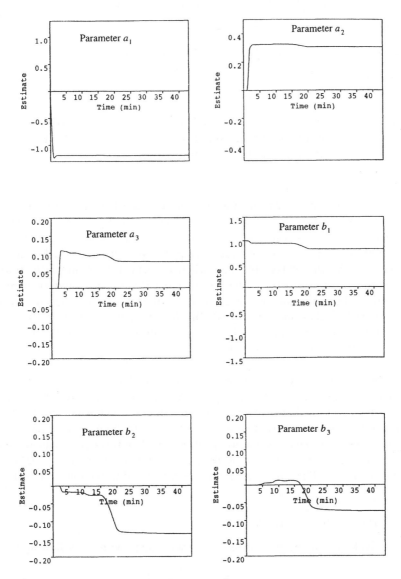

Figure 2.14b System parameter estimates corresponding to Figure 2.14a.

of 7.5 mg and 2.5 mg respectively in order to bring the EMG level down to approximately 15%. At Mark 3, the closed-loop control mode was entered with the fixed PI controller allowed to run for 30 minutes, after which the self-adaptive GPC took over at Mark 4. Both control modes succeeded in keeping a remarkably steady level of paralysis with hardly any fluctuations at all, but looking at the infusion rate plot the period corresponding to the GPC protocol was steadier. Finally at Mark 5 the controller was switched off and the blockade reversed at Mark 6. Notice the return to a 100% baseline suggesting that no unnecessary drug had been administered and that little drift in the relaxation calibration level occurred. Figure 2.14b illustrates the variations of the parameter estimates which were steady for this trial. They finally converged to the following values:

$$\hat{a}_1 = -1.1926 \quad \hat{a}_2 = 0.3059 \quad \hat{a}_3 = 0.0745$$
$$\hat{b}_1 = 0.8109 \quad \hat{b}_2 = -0.1358 \quad \hat{b}_3 = -0.0740$$

These correspond to the following pole/zero positions in the z-plane:

zeros: $0.3972; -0.2297$

poles: $(0.6702 \pm 0.2342\,i); -0.1478$

with an estimated open-loop gain of 3.20. The presence of a pair of complex poles which does not reflect the compartmental idea is probably due to the lack of proper excitation necessary for the identification routine.

Patient 4

During this particular experiment, the subject, a young female, demonstrated very low sensitivity to the muscle relaxant drug. Indeed, as the EMG recording in Figure 2.15 shows, the patient was insensitive to the first bolus dose of 9 mg intravenously administered at Mark 2. Another 2 mg, then 3 mg were given at Mark 3 and Mark 4 respectively. At this stage, the anaesthetist decided to commence automatic control of the infusion at Mark 5 with the fixed PI controller allowed to run only for 5 minutes. The infusion rate of atracurium at 500 μg ml^{-1} began at approximately 60 ml h^{-1} then increased gradually to 80 ml h^{-1}, but even that did not cause the EMG to drop below the 50% line. However, when the GPC took over at Mark ($\bar{5}$), with a combination of (1, 10, 1, 0) for (N_1, N_2, NU, λ) and $T(z^{-1}) = (1 - 0.95\,z^{-1})^2$, it was quick to drive the EMG level to the target in spite of the noise level estimated at $\pm 3\%$ persistently disturbing the output. The controller behaved rather well by rejecting these disturbances and produced a control signal, illustrated on the lower trace of the same figure, which was reasonably active. Undoubtedly, the use of a slower root in the $T(z^{-1})$ polynomial made the controller more robust. The parameter estimation routine, which in this case assumed a second-order model with a one minute time delay, used filtered incremental data for the measurement vector. The parameter estimates converged to the following values:

$$\hat{a}_1 = -1.7674 \quad \hat{a}_2 = 0.7717$$
$$\hat{b}_1 = 0.0471 \quad \hat{b}_2 = -0.0386$$

This is equivalent to a continuous second-order system with the following gain and time constants:

$$\widehat{Gain} = 1.97 \quad \widehat{TC}_1 = 4.19 \text{ min} \quad \widehat{TC}_2 = 48.88 \text{ min}$$

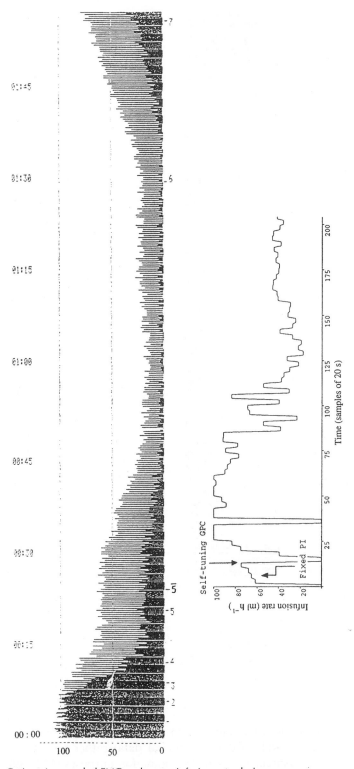

Figure 2.15 Patient 4: recorded EMG and pump infusion rate during surgery.

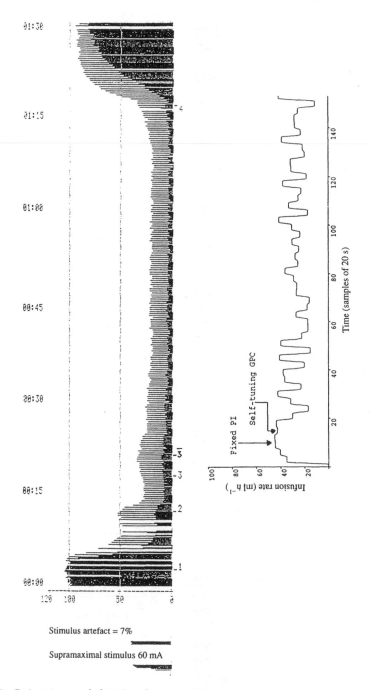

Figure 2.16   Patient 8: recorded EMG and pump infusion rate during surgery.

Before describing the remaining six clinical trials, it is worth noting that throughout the following, full-valued data (positional data) rather than incremental data were used in the measurement vector for estimation purposes. Although this would seem to contradict the idea of an integrative model, it was found to give satisfactory performances as the following results will demonstrate. Parameter estimation assumed a second-order model with a minimum time delay of 1 minute unless otherwise specified, and initial conditions included a covariance matrix and a forgetting factor of $Cov = 10^2 . I$ and $\rho = 0.995$ respectively. Parameter estimates were initialised so as to reflect a continuous second-order system with the following gain and time constants:

$$\theta_i = [1.15, 0.34 \text{ min}, 16.13 \text{ min}]$$

Patient 8

After bolus doses of 8 mg then 3 mg administered at Mark 1 and Mark 2 respectively on the upper trace of Figure 2.16 (again suggesting a low sensitivity patient), the loop was closed at Mark (3) when the EMG level reached approximately 28%. The PI was allowed to run for 5 minutes and produced an overshoot of 12%. When the GPC took over at Mark ($\bar{3}$) assuming a combination of (1, 30, 1, 5) for (N_1, N_2, NU, λ) and no filter, it was quick to reduce the overshoot by making the EMG track efficiently the 20% target. The control signal, whose variations are shown on the lower trace of the same figure, was good and reasonably active.

Patient 9

This experiment was the longest in the series of trials. The subject, a young male, underwent a three-hour surgery requiring muscle relaxation. Mark 1 on the trace of Figure 2.17 is the time at which suxamethonium was administered before the trachea was intubated. A return to the 100% EMG level was achieved at Mark 4 when a large bolus dose of muscle relaxant drug of 24 mg was given intravenously, and this completely wiped out the EMG tracing, which only started to reappear again 12 minutes later. At Mark 5 the automatic control mode was entered with the PI controller providing initial control for 30 minutes until Mark 6. At this time the GPC took over with the same controller and estimation parameters as before, except that instead of assuming a minimum delay of 1 minute, the $B(z^{-1})$ polynomial structure was extended by one coefficient to absorb this value. Initial conditions for the estimates were taken to be:

$$\hat{a}_1 = -0.9927$$
$$\hat{a}_2 = 0.0496$$
$$\hat{b}_1 = 0.0$$
$$\hat{b}_2 = 0.0471$$
$$\hat{b}_3 = 0.0183$$

These were chosen to reflect the same gain, time constants, and time delay as in the previous case.

At Mark 7 the control had to be switched off due to a lack of computer disk space. From then on, the anaesthetist had to resume manual control with bolus doses of 10 mg each at times indicated by Mark 8 and Mark 9. The large fluctuations in the EMG level during this phase indicate the difficulty of manual control via bolus injections. At Mark 10 the blockade was reversed with neostigmine. As shown in the same figure, the PI controller induced an 8% overshoot followed by a

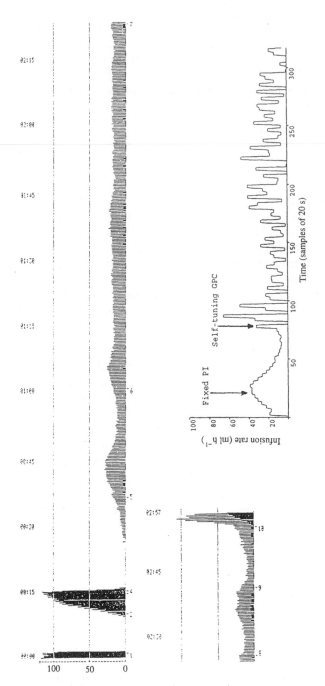

Figure 2.17   Patient 9: recorded EMG and pump infusion rate during surgery.

10% undershoot of the EMG level, but this was quickly eliminated as soon as the GPC took over. The EMG level was quite steady, fluctuating between 17% and 20% leading to a highly activated control signal as the lower trace of the same figure illustrates, this occurring in spite of the relatively large value of the output horizon and the non-zero control weighting sequence. Parameter estimates suggest indeed a value of time delay greater than or equal to 1 minute, since $\hat{b}_1$ was an insignificant value. These parameter estimates converged to the following final values:

$$\hat{a}_1 = -1.0149 \quad \hat{a}_2 = 0.0284$$

$$\hat{b}_1 = 0.0048 \quad \hat{b}_2 = 0.0228 \quad \hat{b}_3 = 0.0353$$

This is equivalent to a continuous second-order system with the following gain and time constants:

$$\widehat{\text{Gain}} = 4.66 \quad \widehat{TC}_1 = 0.28 \text{ min} \quad \widehat{TC}_2 = 71.44 \text{ min}$$

These values suggest a high sensitivity patient with a slow dominant time constant.

2.6.4 Analysis of the data

In order to analyse the data, three indices were used: the mean value, the standard deviation (SD), and the root mean square deviation (RMSD). These last two indices are commonly used to give an indication of the spread of a set of values around the mean value and the target value respectively. They are defined together with the mean by the following two formulae:

$$\text{Mean} = \bar{X} = \sum_{i=1}^{N} X_i \tag{2.27}$$

$$\text{SD} = \sqrt{\frac{1}{N} \sum (X_i - \bar{X})^2} \tag{2.28}$$

where X_i and N are the current measurement, and the total number of points considered respectively, and

$$\text{RMSD} = \sqrt{\frac{1}{N} \sum (X_i - \text{TRGT})^2} \tag{2.29}$$

where X_i is as defined previously and TRGT is the reference target. Table 2.3 summarises these values for each of the ten patients in the trial.

The mean value of $T1\%$ for each patient was calculated for those trials where closed-loop infusion was started when $T1\%$ returned to 15% after administration of the initial bolus dose of atracurium (patients 3, 6, 9 and 10). For those experiments where closed-loop control was initiated earlier, the mean was evaluated from the moment $T1\%$ crossed the target point for the first time. As shown in Table 2.3, the mean values of $T1\%$ suggest that the degree of neuromuscular blockade obtained with the ten patients was very satisfactory. Maximum overshoots were recorded with patients 7 (22%), 9 (8%), 1 (7%) and 6 (7%). This relates to the wrong time at which the closed-loop mode was entered. Indeed, with patient 7, automatic control was operational when $T1$ reached 19% after recovery from the bolus, and the pre-loaded PI controller value for PL was not large enough to shorten the stabilisation period. This is probably the biggest problem facing such a controller because it is not always possible to switch to automatic control at $T1 = 15\%$ as experiments with patients 1, 2, 4, 5 and 8 have demonstrated. These patients had very low sensitivity to the drug, so that even large bolus doses did not induce the expected drop in

Table 2.3 Summary of each patient's data

Patient	Total points	Mean $T1\%$	SD (%)	RMSD (%)
1*	197	17.50	4.13	4.83
2*	58	19.92	1.36	1.37
3*	134	19.43	2.56	2.63
4*	123	18.49	3.51	3.82
5*	97	21.85	1.76	2.56
6*	94	21.59	3.57	3.91
7*	387	20.14	6.89	6.89
8*	99	20.29	1.02	1.07
9	318	18.42	3.31	3.67
10**	66	16.91	2.64	3.26

* 20% $T1$ target.
** 15% $T1$ target.

the EMG baseline. One solution to this problem of initial overshoot is, of course, to switch to the self-adaptive GPC a lot sooner, as was the case for patients 8 and 10 which both produced a mean $T1\%$ level close to the target, i.e. 20.29% (SD 1.02) and 16.91% (SD 2.64) respectively. Perhaps more justice would have been done to the self-adaptive GPC, as far as Table 2.3 is concerned, if its corresponding values were evaluated only during the period GPC was operating, since all the bigger overshoots were induced by the PI controller. Obviously, the initiation of the self-tuning GPC at an earlier stage could be detrimental due to the fact that the estimator would not have gathered enough information about the patient to ensure adequate control. This may therefore produce a poor performance, especially if the wrong filter is used in the case of incremental data for the measurement vector. The use of positional data in this case would be advantageous. This has been demonstrated in the last 6 experiments, and particularly during the trial with patient 10 where in spite of the use of the operating point being close to the nonlinear region (15% $T1$ target) (Mahfouf et al., 1992), the controller behaved sensibly by producing a good response and a reasonably active control. Table 2.3 also shows that the RMSD as well as the SD values were relatively low for all patients, except those of patient 7 which reached a value of SD = RMSD = ± 6.89. However, these values include the case where the concentration was doubled halfway through the run, meaning that the pump should drive at approximately half speed but had to wait for the effect of the previous higher infusions to wear off. For patient 1, the RMSD and SD values were outside the 4% range (4.83% and 4.13% respectively) due to the wrong choice of the filter $T(z^{-1})$ order, although otherwise the performance was good.

Regarding the infusion rate variations for the ten patients, an analysis of the mean atracurium drug consumption per minute and per kilogram body weight was performed, allowing for the corresponding muscle relaxant drug concentration. Table 2.4 summarises this evaluation.

As shown in Table 2.4, the highest dose of muscle relaxant drug was recorded with patient 4 (6.81 μg kg^{-1} min^{-1}) who had a relatively low gain (1.97). The lowest drug doses were those for patients 3 and 2, where the GPC algorithm used the filter polynomial $T(z^{-1})$ which, as already seen, reduces the overall feedback gain leading to smoother control actions. The mean dose consumed by patient 7 was surprisingly

Table 2.4 Summary of each patient's drug consumption dose

Patient	Total points	Mean dose (μg kg^{-1} min^{-1})	SD
1*	197	6.65	2.35
2*	58	2.65	0.07
3**	134	1.57	0.28
4**	123	6.81	2.78
5*	97	6.77	1.64
6*	94	5.27	2.39
7***	387	5.38	4.43
8*	99	6.34	1.75
9*	318	4.03	2.98
10**	66	5.30	1.81

* 1000 μg ml^{-1} concentration.
** 500 μg ml^{-1} concentration.
*** both concentrations used.

low at 5.38 μg kg^{-1} min^{-1} considering the high control signal activity. Despite the severe concentration change made during this trial, the algorithm performed well. With this latter trial full-valued data were used for the estimator, and no filter was included to compensate for any unmodelled dynamics and to reduce high frequency components.

A summary of the results for the first nine patients is given in Table 2.5 where the mean and SD indices are displayed for the duration of automatic control, mean drug dose consumption, the mean, RMSD and the SD. The last experiment was excluded since the 15% target was different from the other trials.

The value of 3.12% for the mean of standard deviation of $T1$ indicates that, generally, a steady level of blockade was obtained. Moreover, the fact that this value was so close to the value of the mean of the root-mean square deviation of $T1$ (3.41%) implies that the degree of neuromuscular blockade was close to the target. The value 19.74% as the mean value of mean of $T1$% reinforces the argument that the individual $T1$% values were also close to the target. At this stage it is too soon to draw any conclusions about a clear correlation between the patient's reaction to the initial bolus and the overall control performance. Suffice to say that for the three control modes used (manual, fixed controller, self-adaptive), the self-adaptive scheme proved the most robust and efficient. Moreover, the mean dose of muscle relaxant drug (5.05 μg kg^{-1} min^{-1}) was far lower than that which would be obtained by anaesthetists using bolus doses, and certainly lower than the range recommended by the manufacturers of atracurium.

Table 2.5 Summary of patients' data ($n = 9$)

Parameter	Mean	SD	Range
Automatic control duration (min)	62.33	33.04	30–130
Dose (μg kg^{-1} min^{-1})	5.05	1.80	1.57–6.81
Mean of $T1$ (%)	19.74	1.37	17.50–21.85
RMSD of $T1$ (%)	3.41	1.69	1.07–6.89
SD of $T1$ (%)	3.12	1.68	1.02–6.89

2.7 Conclusions

The application of self-adaptive GPC to on-line control of muscle relaxation has been successful in achieving two primary goals. These are the maintaining of a steady level of paralysis with minimum deviation from set-point, and the reduction of total muscle relaxant dosage. The algorithm has proved to be robust with respect to external disturbances, such as heavy electrical interference from surgical diathermy. This is particularly important since operating theatres are 'electrically dirty' environments. The overall computer control system proved to be easy to manage, with most of the clinical trials being performed without the presence of an engineer. Anaesthetics gained confidence in the controller as the trials proceeded and the system demonstrated good response, particularly in the case of low sensitivity patients where the bolus doses were clearly inadequate at the beginning of the operation. They were amenable to implementing changes in the design parameters of the GPC algorithm, providing that these were explained to them clearly and rationally. Throughout the work it was emphasised that the closed-loop regulation was an assistance to the anaesthetist, relieving him of tedium during normal periods of operation and enabling him to concentrate on the higher-level supervisory control aspects for which no form of automation could be envisaged. The ability of adaptive GPC to cope with massively varying patient parameters, particularly relating to gain changes, has been demonstrated in the clinical trials.

From a design viewpoint, GPC offers considerable flexibility for goal-achievement via its 'tuning knobs'. This has been exploited extensively in this work via simulation studies. In addition to off-line selection of design parameters via a SUN workstation, the prior validation of the total systems software via on-line microcomputer-based simulations significantly reduced the initial time required to achieve successful clinical experiments. Several aspects of GPC were explored during the trials, one of which was the use of full-valued data for the estimation rather than incremental ones. Although the effect of eliminating the offset from the data is absent, the estimates obtained were consistent and little biased, a problem which could certainly have occurred with purely incremental data and wrong filter choice.

Consideration of the best settings for the GPC design parameters obtained from the simulations and trials leads to the following conclusions. If full-valued data are being used for the measurement vector, then values of $(1, 20, 1, 5)$ for (N_1, N_2, NU, λ) were found to be appropriate. Conversely, for incremental data, values of $(1, 10, 1, 0)$ for (N_1, N_2, NU, λ) together with a second-order filter having slow roots of the form $T(z^{-1}) = (1 - 0.95\,z^{-1})^2$ were found to be desirable.

CHAPTER THREE

Propofol Induced Anaesthesia: a Comparative Control Study Using a Derived Nonlinear Model

3.1 Introduction

Propofol is an intravenous anaesthetic agent which has gained considerable popularity over other agents such as thiopentone. This popularity is justified by some of its properties such as its good solubility, short onset time, and quick recovery. It is suitable for both induction and maintenance of anaesthesia, and the blood levels of propofol (2.5 to 6 μg ml^{-1}) required for surgery have been reported widely (Schuttler *et al.*, 1988; White and Kenny, 1990). The knowledge of these levels, together with the well-known difficulties associated with quantifying anaesthesia, have encouraged the use of a pharmacokinetic model-driven infusion system to deliver propofol at a continuous infusion for the maintenance of anaesthesia.

Workers have characterised propofol's pharmacokinetic parameters and used these values within computer programs to administer the drug according to target concentration infusion (TCI) (White and Kenny, 1990) or computer assisted infusion (CAI) (Schuttler *et al.*, 1988) schemes rather than as simple manual infusions for maintenance of anaesthesia. Following a bolus injection, whole blood propofol concentration decreases very rapidly due to distribution of the drug. Using a three-compartment model half-lives have been estimated as follows: $T_{1/2\,\alpha} = 2$ min, $T_{1/2\,\beta} = 50$–60 min, $T_{1/2\,\gamma} = 6$–12 h (Kirkpatrick *et al.*, 1988). The high clearance of propofol (1.5 to 2 l min^{-1}) also ensures minimal residual sedative effect during the recovery period despite the long elimination half-life which is indicative of the slow return of propofol back to the central compartment from a deep compartment with limited perfusion.

Great interest is also being shown in using the pharmacodynamic effects of drugs to control administration of drugs by such CAI schemes, but these involve identification and measurement of appropriate effects. Propofol is principally a hypnotic drug with no analgesic properties. EEG and evoked response effects have been proposed as a measure of anaesthetic effect (Shafer *et al.*, 1988) but at the present time there is no single measure which is accepted as standard and the hardware required is not generally available in theatres.

The success behind TCI or CAI systems is mainly attributed to the fact that despite the nature of the controller which is model-driven and does not include any measurement, the user, in this case the anaesthetist, utilises some kind of true feedback when the target plasma concentrations are allowed to change on-line, and this is based on noticeable, vital signs that can be seen with the patient such as sweating, movements, etc. In other words, the drug *effect* is used as an *implicit* criterion in order to adjust the propofol infusion rates.

As with all anaesthetic agents, cardiovascular effects also accompany the use of propofol and these have been analysed following its use for both induction and maintenance of anaesthesia (Tackley *et al.*, 1989; Peacock *et al.*, 1990). The most prominent effect of propofol is a reduction in arterial pressure during induction of anaesthesia. In the absence of cardiovascular disease and premedicant drugs, an induction dose of propofol will result in 25–40% reduction in systolic arterial pressures with similar changes in mean and diastolic pressures. This decrease may be associated with a decrease in cardiac output and it is worth noting that during maintenance of anaesthesia with propofol infusion, systolic arterial pressure remains 20–30% below pre-induction values.

Although the arterial pressure changes are not a measure of anaesthetic depth, they are an important inferential factor in determining depth of anaesthesia and in patient safety. Previous work has been carried out using arterial pressure measurements to adjust the concentration of the inhalational agent isoflurane via a computer controlled vaporiser (Robb *et al.*, 1993; Meier *et al.*, 1992). This consideration represents the main motivation behind the present study whose purpose is to outline the problems associated with the strategy based on drug pharmacokinetics, and also to show how the propofol pharmacokinetic model can be extended to include pharmacodynamics and hence, allow the design and development of a feedback control strategy able to realise effective regulation. The measurable variable in this case is Mean Arterial Pressure (MAP), considered to be a useful indicator of depth of anaesthesia (Kirkpatrick *et al.*, 1988; Shafer *et al.*, 1988; Tackley *et al.*, 1989).

3.2 Pharmacokinetic model for propofol

The disposition of infused propofol is assumed to be described by an equation representing a linear three-compartment model as Figure 3.1 illustrates. Following a propofol injection u into the central compartment (1), elimination and inter-compartmental distribution can be defined by the following system equations:

$$\begin{cases} \dot{x}_1 = k_{21}x_2 + k_{31}x_3 - k_{12}x_1 - k_{13}x_1 - k_{10}x_1 + u \\ \dot{x}_2 = k_{12}x_1 - k_{21}x_2 \\ \dot{x}_3 = k_{13}x_1 - k_{31}x_3 \end{cases} \qquad (3.1)$$

where x_i is the amount of drug in compartment i at time t, x_i is the change of drug amount in compartment i, k_{ij} $(i \neq j \neq 0)$ is the rate constant governing the drug transfer from compartment i to compartment j, and k_{10} is the rate of elimination.

Using Laplace transforms leads to the following transfer function between the

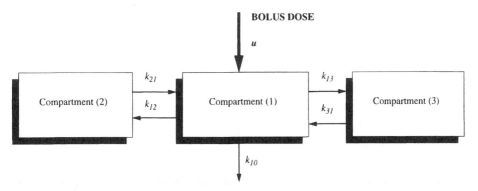

Figure 3.1 Diagram representing the three-compartment model associated with propofol.

drug input and the central compartment drug amount:

$$\frac{X_1(s)}{U(s)} = \frac{s^2 + (k_{21} + k_{31})s + k_{21}k_{31}}{s^3 + pp_1s^2 + pp_2 s + pp_3} \tag{3.2}$$

where

$$X_i(s) = L(x_i), \; U(s) = L(u) \qquad L: \text{Laplace operator}$$

$$pp_1 = k_{31} + k_{21} + k_{12} + k_{13} + k_{10}$$

$$pp_2 = k_{21}k_{31} + k_{12}k_{31} + k_{13}k_{21} + k_{10}k_{31} + k_{10}k_{21}$$

$$pp_3 = k_{21}k_{31}k_{10}$$

Hence, the plasma concentration can be obtained by dividing X_1 by V_c where V_c is the central compartment volume.

As mentioned earlier, several studies have been conducted in which data for the microconstants of rate of transfer between the three compartments have been evaluated (Gepts *et al.*, 1987, 1988; Marsh *et al.*, 1991). However, throughout this study only the data used by Marsh and co-workers, which are slightly modified from those of Gepts *et al.*, will be considered. Hence, substituting these values in equation (3.2) leads to the following transfer function:

$$G(s) = \frac{X_1(s)}{U(s)} = \frac{s^2 + q_1s + q_2}{s^3 + pp_1s^2 + pp_2 s + pp_3} \tag{3.3}$$

where

$$q_1 = 0.0583 \; \text{min}^{-1}$$

$$q_2 = 0.0001815 \; \text{min}^{-2}$$

$$pp_1 = 0.3312 \; \text{min}^{-1}$$

$$pp_2 = 0.0097933 \; \text{min}^{-2}$$

$$pp_3 = 0.0000215985 \; \text{min}^{-3}$$

Equation (3.3) can also be written in the following 'time-constant' form:

$$G(s) = \frac{K_1(1 + T_{c5} s)(1 + T_{c6} s)}{(1 + T_{c1}s)(1 + T_{c2} s)(1 + T_{c3} s)} \tag{3.4}$$

where

$K_1 = 8.4034$ min

$T_{c1} = 3.3484$ min

$T_{c2} = 33.1663$ min

$T_{c3} = 416.9103$ min

$T_{c5} = 18.1818$ min

$T_{c6} = 303.0303$ min

Runge–Kutta fourth-order, Tustin and zero-order hold methods can be used for simulating equation (3.4). The first method was adopted throughout this study. Therefore, using this method, equation (3.4) allows one to monitor the movement of drug through various compartments for a bolus dose of propofol administered at 200 mg min^{-1} for 30 seconds. Figure 3.2 shows the theoretical plasma concentration (compartment 1) against time which peaked at a concentration value of 6.12 μg ml^{-1} at time 0.50 min for a 67 kg patient, before falling again according to the exponential phases corresponding to the three constants T_{c1}, T_{c2} and T_{c3}. The same figure also shows the drug concentrations in compartments 2 and 3 respectively.

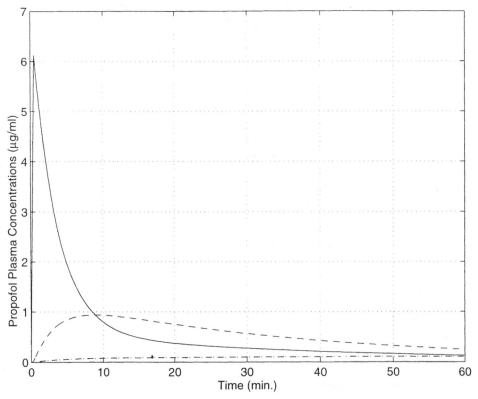

Figure 3.2 Open-loop responses corresponding to the compartmental concentrations when a bolus size of 200 mg min^{-1} of propofol is administered for 30 seconds to a 67 kg patient: solid line – central compartment concentration; dashed line – second compartment concentration; dashdot line – third compartment concentration.

At this stage it is worth mentioning that the knowledge provided by equation (3.4) in terms of plasma concentration levels associated with particular drug inputs plays a crucial role in determining the propofol dose at which an acceptable anaesthetic state can be achieved and sustained. As already mentioned, although such levels have now been established and shown to work in many cases (Schuttler *et al.*, 1988; Tackley *et al.*, 1989; Marsh *et al.*, 1991), the relationship between depth of anaesthesia and propofol inputs will remain an open subject as long as no direct single *reliable* measurement for depth of anaesthesia is available. At this stage we believe that the *rapprochement* between the two can be narrowed by an inferential variable directly related to propofol and which could provide one with some measure of depth of anaesthesia. This has prompted us to model the cardiovascular pharmacodynamics associated with this drug as described in the following section.

3.3 Automatic infusion of propofol based on pharmacokinetics and its problems

3.3.1 Modified Alvis algorithm

A protocol used for controlling drug infusions was first introduced by Alvis and coworkers (Alvis *et al.*, 1985) who controlled fentanyl infusion during anaesthesia employing a method which was later to be modified by Jannett (1986) and Maitre *et al.* (1986). The key to the method lies in keeping the plasma level constant at the desired concentration. In order to achieve this the right infusion rate has to be determined. Once the desired concentration is reached and maintained at that precise level, the system is said to be functioning in open-loop. If the anaesthetist, however, decides to decrease or increase the plasma level, the whole system must switch to the mode known as the model closed-loop mode (referred to here as pseudo closed-loop mode) and the new infusion rate has to be calculated. It is worth noting that all calculations are done assuming a patient model whose pharmacokinetic parameters are those which are thought to represent the average pharmacokinetic profile of a certain group of patients. The following sections endeavour to outline the various steps involved in the algorithm depending on the control mode.

In open-loop conditions

The propofol concentration in the central compartment is to be kept constant, i.e. $\dot{x}_1(t) = 0$, or $x_1(t) =$ constant for $t > 0$. Initially, all compartments in Figure 3.1 have a propofol concentration of 0. In order to achieve a certain target concentration in the central compartment with a volume V_c, sufficient drug must be given as a single dose. Because the central compartment concentration is to be kept constant the amount of propofol entering it must be equal to the amount of propofol leaving it. The drug leaves the blood to pass into volumes 2 and 3 at a gradually decreasing rate as their respective concentrations increase. The drug is also metabolised in the liver at a clearance rate ($k_{10} V_c$). Therefore, the infusion rate function $u'(t)$ must be equal to the rate of elimination plus the rate of distribution to the peripheral compartments. After development it follows that:

$$u'(t) = C_c V_c (k_{10} + k_{12} e^{-k_{21}t} + k_{13} e^{-k_{31}t}) \tag{3.5}$$

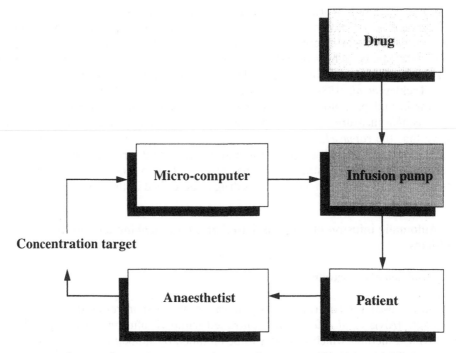

Figure 3.3   Schematic diagram representing the control system used by Alvis *et al.* (1985).

where

V_c = volume of central compartment (litres)

C_c = concentration of drug in the central compartment (μg l^{-1})

In pseudo closed-loop conditions

At the start of this mode the program operates in the open-loop mode rapidly trying to maintain the desired plasma level. It remains functional under these conditions until the clinician decides to change the target plasma concentration. Once the new value to be targeted is acknowledged, the program chooses a path that depends very much upon the value of the new concentration NC_c with reference to the current concentration C_c, i.e. if $NC_c = C_c$, $NC_c > C_c$ or $NC_c < C_c$.

1. $NC_c > C_c$

$$u'(t) = V_c(NC_c k_{10} + (NC_c - C_{20})k_{12} e^{-k_{21}t} + (NC_c - C_{30})k_{13} e^{-k_{31}t}) \tag{3.6}$$

where t is reset to 0 after the loading dose is infused and C_{20} and C_{30} are the drug concentrations in the peripheral compartments at the time of the change in the set-point plasma level. Let the following be the various steps involved in the derivation of the concentrations in the second and third compartments. The concentrations in the peripheral compartments can be derived by developing equation (3.1)

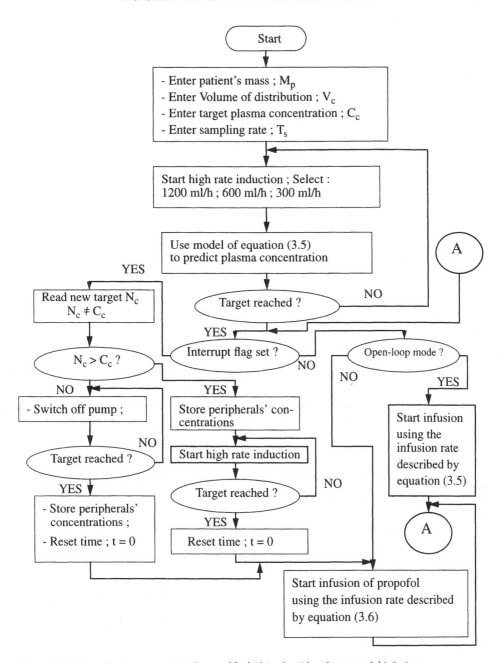

Figure 3.4 Flow chart summarising the modified Alvis algorithm for propofol infusion.

and by using the following system identity (Jacobs *et al.*, 1990):

$$V_2 = V_c \frac{k_{12}}{k_{21}}$$
$$V_3 = V_c \frac{k_{13}}{k_{31}}$$

(3.7)

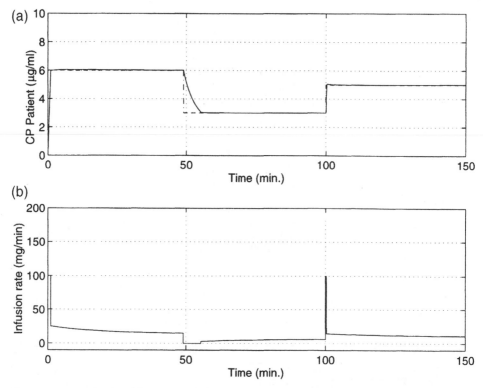

Figure 3.5 Pseudo closed-loop control of propofol infusion using the modified Alvis algorithm in the nominal case. (a) Solid line: patient's plasma concentration (CP); dashdot line: target. (b) Infusion rate profile.

where V_i, $i = 2, 3$ is the volume of the ith compartment. It follows, therefore, that in terms of concentrations equation (3.7) becomes:

$$C_2 = C_1 \frac{k_{21}}{s + k_{21}}$$
$$C_3 = C_1 \frac{k_{31}}{s + k_{31}}$$

(3.8)

where C_i ($i = 2, 3$) is the drug concentration associated with the ith compartment.

2. $NC_c = C_c$ The program operates in open-loop and no change in the infusion is required.

3. $NC_c < C_c$ The infusion rate is set to zero to allow the plasma level to decrease as a result of elimination and redistribution. Once the plasma level has reached the new target concentration NC_c the time 't' is reset to 0 and the infusion is restarted according to equation (3.6); C_{20} and C_{30} are the peripherals' concentrations at the time of the infusion restart.

Figure 3.3 is a schematic diagram which represents the overall control system and Figure 3.4 is a flow chart outlining the various steps involved in the overall open-loop and pseudo closed-loop control protocol.

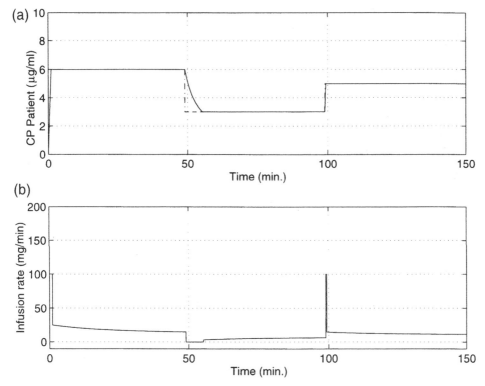

Figure 3.6 Generalised predictive control (GPC) of propofol infusion in the nominal case. (a) Solid line: patient's plasma concentration (CP); dashdot line: target. (b) Infusion rate profile.

3.3.2 The GPC algorithm

The algorithm is similar to the one described in Chapter 2, Section 2.4 by equations (2.9) to (2.20).

3.3.3 Simulation results

The simulation study consisted of using both the above control strategies on the model described in Section 3.2. The model of equation (3.4) was simulated using a Runge–Kutta fourth-order numerical routine with an integration interval of 1/60 and a sampling time of 1 second; this was judged adequate to track the drug movement sufficiently quickly. The set-point command was 6 μg ml^{-1} until sample time 50 min, then 3 μg ml^{-1} until sample time 100 min, and finally 5 μg ml^{-1} until sample time 150 min where the controller was switched off. It is worth noting that in the case of the modified Alvis algorithm, and in order to reach the initial plasma concentration as fast as possible, it is advisable to start the infusion at a high rate (100 mg min^{-1} in this study) until the predicted plasma (central compartment) concentration reaches the target within a user-defined tolerance. In the GPC case, a combination of (1, 10, 4, 0) was used for the tuning knobs (N_1, N_2, NU, λ) respectively. In addition, the algorithm used the parameter estimates calculated from the discretised model of equation (3.4) with 3 as and 3 bs at a sampling rate of 1 second. Figures 3.5 and 3.6 show how both protocols displayed excellent properties in open-

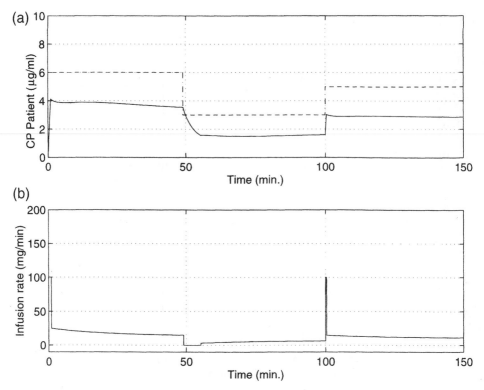

Figure 3.7 Pseudo closed-loop control of propofol infusion using the modified Alvis algorithm in the mismatch case, the nominal case. (a) Solid line: patient's plasma concentration (CP); dashdot line: target. (b) Infusion rate profile.

loop and pseudo closed-loop modes. Next, an experiment was conducted in which a mismatch between the model parameters and those of the patient was simulated. The result of the run is shown in Figure 3.7 where for the modified Alvis the performance degraded.

Since the modified Alvis algorithm cannot inherently use any measurement, it is believed that if a measurement was available to the fixed GPC algorithm, the performance would certainly have improved. On the question of measurements, it would be interesting to use an inferential variable related to propofol and which could provide some measurement of depth of anaesthesia. As mentioned in Section 3.1, cardiovascular system effects of propofol suggest that there is a 25% to 40% reduction in mean arterial pressure (MAP) after an induction dose of propofol of a certain size. Therefore, in the next section, an attempt is made at modelling the pharmacodynamics of propofol with respect to MAP.

3.4   Pharmacodynamics associated with propofol

Before further investigations are made, two important questions need to be addressed sequentially:

1. Can we speculate about a hypothetical compartment which is related to the central compartment and which contains an amount of drug?

2. Is there any relationship between such a compartment concentration, or the plasma concentration, and the actual effect of the drug which in this case is the change in mean arterial pressure (Δ MAP)?

Before answering the first question it is vital to establish the kind of relationship that exists between the plasma concentration and Δ MAP. In order to do that, blood pressure measurements were taken from a study conducted on 60 consenting patients in theatre following a clearly defined infusion protocol (Peacock et al., 1990). Using the same protocol on the average pharmacokinetics model of equation (3.4) (fourth-order Runge–Kutta integration method with a 1 second sampling interval) the various plasma concentrations were calculated for each of the 60 patients. The following sections review the methods and the results obtained.

3.4.1 Patients and method for determining blood pressure measurements

The study conducted by Peacock and co-workers (Peacock et al., 1990) considered 60 elderly patients to establish the effect of different rates of infusion of propofol for induction of anaesthesia. At this stage it must be stressed that it is not the objective of this present investigation to confirm any conclusions the previous authors might have drawn following their study. Hence, only 10 from the above 60 patients were selected for our investigation, the criterion for selection being the infusion regime which involved a minimal number of incremental changes in the rate of propofol administration.

All patients underwent body surface or urological surgery lasting between half to one hour. Patients with a history of significant medical disease were excluded from the investigation. All patients were given fentanyl 0.75 μg kg^{-1} i.v. 5 minutes before induction of anaesthesia. For induction of anaesthesia they were given propofol at 50, 100 or 200 mg min^{-1} for a period varying between 45 and 135 seconds until loss of consciousness. A propofol infusion administered at 0.10 mg kg^{-1} min^{-1} was used to maintain anaesthesia. This infusion was altered according to clinical requirements as judged by patient movements or cardiovascular responses and any alterations were recorded. Arterial pressure was measured using a Dinamap instrument. Cardiovascular measurements were made before and 4 minutes after administration of fentanyl, at the end of induction, and at 2 minutes, 5 minutes and at 5 minute intervals thereafter during maintenance of anaesthesia. Table 3.1 gives details of the three groups of patients considered for investigation.

3.4.2 Method for determining the corresponding plasma concentrations

As already mentioned, because it is practically impossible to obtain on-line plasma concentration measurements we used a fourth-order Runge–Kutta integration method on equation (3.4) with a sampling interval of 1 second and calculated the central compartment concentrations for each patient after the induction phase, and at 2, 5, 10, 15 and 20 minutes later, leading altogether to 6 data points. In some

Table 3.1 Table representing the details of experiments for the three groups of patients considered

Induction rate (mg min^{-1})	n	Age (yr) (mean)	Weight (kg) (mean)	Induction dose (mg kg^{-1}) (mean)	Induction time (min) (mean)
50	1	74	60	1.32	1.58
100	4	76	65.3	1.59	1.04
200	5	69	71	2.65	0.94

instances these were reduced to 5 data points if a particular blood pressure measurement was judged to be erroneous.

3.4.3 Results of experiments

Combining the data provided by the experiments above and those obtained following the simulation runs conducted previously, Figure 3.8 shows a sample from the responses obtained, where the changes in mean arterial pressure (mmHg) are plotted against the corresponding calculated plasma concentrations (μg ml^{-1}). The plot, similar to all the other plots, showed an underlying trend which suggests that as the plasma concentration decreases the change in mean arterial pressure increases, which is not clinically justified. This observation seems to support the fact that the

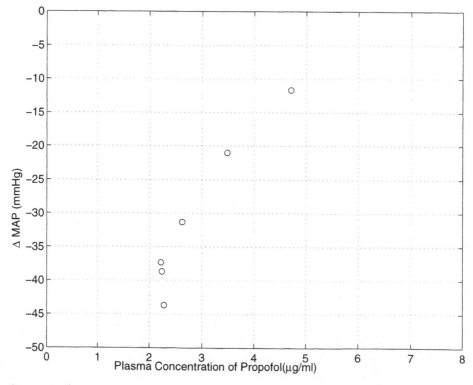

Figure 3.8 Plasma concentration (CP) versus change of mean arterial pressure Δ MAP.

time course of some drug effects does not parallel the time course of drug computed to reside in the central compartment. This phenomenon is usually referred to as 'kinetic-dynamic dissociation' and the necessary modelling extension is commonly called effect-compartment modelling. Effect-compartment modelling consists of including an additional compartment in the classical three-compartment structure. This so-called effect compartment is assumed to receive a vanishingly small mass of drug (so as not to affect the time course of drug disposition in the rest of the model) at a rate directly proportional to the central compartment drug concentration ($k_{1E} \ll$) (Sheiner et al., 1979). The drug exits this effect compartment in accordance with another rate constant k_{E0} (see Figure 3.9) which is determined using the technique described in the next section.

3.4.4 Method for determining the microconstant k_{E0}

In order to obtain an approximate value of this constant we used the observation that after two minutes the effect-compartment concentration should approximately be around 40% of the maximal or final value. In light of this consideration we establish first the expression associated with the effect-compartment concentration, recall equation (3.1):

$$\dot{x}_1 = k_{21}x_2 + k_{31}x_3 - k_{12}x_1 - k_{13}x_1 - k_{10}x_1 + u$$

where

$$\dot{x}_2 = k_{12}x_1 - k_{21}x_2$$
$$\dot{x}_3 = k_{13}x_1 - k_{31}x_3$$

(3.9)

But referring to Figure 3.9 it follows that:

$$\frac{dX_E}{dt} = k_{1e}X_1 - k_{E0}X_E$$

X_E = amount of drug in the effect compartment

k_{1E} is chosen arbitrarily, but smaller than the smallest rate constant in the rest

of the model

Solving for X_E gives:

$$X_E = k_{1E}\frac{X_1}{s + k_{E0}}$$

(3.10)

It should be noted that it is meaningful to relate drug effect to the concentration of drug in plasma, rather than to an amount of drug in the hypothetical effect compartment (Sheiner et al., 1979). It is possible to do so by considering that at steady state there will be a steady-state plasma concentration CP_{ss} and a unique corresponding steady-state X_E. For the effect compartment to reach steady state, its exit rate constant must be greater than zero which is the case for k_{E0}. At steady state no transfer of drug into or out of any compartment occurs, i.e. $dX_E/dt = 0$.

This implies that:

$$k_{1E}X_1 - k_{E0}X_E = 0$$

(3.11)

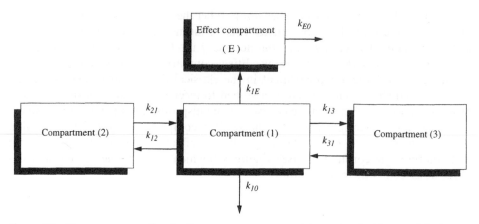

Figure 3.9   Diagram representing the three-compartment model associated with propofol when extended to include the 'effect compartment'.

Hence

$$X_1 = \frac{k_{E0}}{k_{1E}} X_E \qquad (3.12)$$

But the plasma concentration is given by:

$$CP = \frac{X_1}{V_c} \qquad (3.13)$$

However, at steady state:

$$CP_{ss} = \frac{X}{V_c} = \frac{k_{E0}}{k_{1E}} \frac{X_E}{V_c} \qquad (3.14)$$

Finally, using equation (3.10) the plasma concentration is given by the following formula:

$$CP_{ss} = \frac{k_{E0}}{s + k_{E0}} \frac{X_1}{V_c} \qquad (3.15)$$

Notice that in the case of equation (3.15) the rate k_{1E} does not appear and therefore its value is irrelevant. It is also worth noting that expression (3.15) is also used for the effect-compartment concentration $C_e(t)$. Hence, we will refer to it as $C_e(t)$ throughout.

Having established the expression for plasma concentration, the next step involved a trial-and-error operation to find the right microconstant k_{E0}, taking into account the clinical observation that after approximately 2 minutes the effect compartment concentration should approximately be equal to 40% of the maximum effect. After an exhaustive search, which consisted of experimenting with various time constants and observing the time course of the effect-compartment concentration, a value of $k_{E0} = 0.10$ min^{-1} was obtained. Figure 3.10 is a sample response for one of the ten patients considered showing the time course of the plasma concentration at steady state when the above microconstant value was used. In addition, as suggested by Gentry and co-workers (1993), we included a 20 second delay to

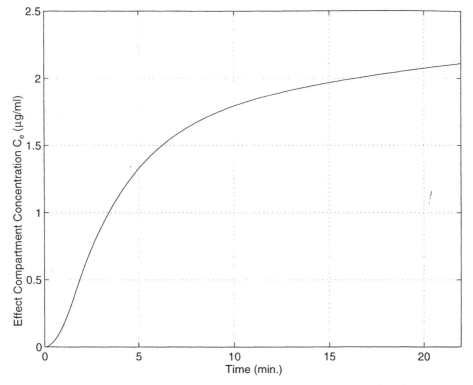

Figure 3.10 Effect compartment concentration (C_e) versus time for $k_{E0} = 0.10 \text{ min}^{-1}$.

account for a mean circulation time for the transport of the drug through the circulation from the arm to the cerebral vessels (Veall and Peacock, 1994). Hence, equation (3.4) becomes:

$$G_2(s) = \frac{X_{Ess}(s)}{U(s)} = G_1(s)\frac{k_{E0}}{s + k_{E0}} e^{-\tau s} \tag{3.16}$$

or

$$G_2(s) = \frac{X_{Ess}(s)}{U(s)} = \frac{K_1(1 + T_{c5} s)(1 + T_{c6} s) e^{-\tau s}}{(1 + T_{c1}s)(1 + T_{c2} s)(1 + T_{c3} s)(1 + T_{c4} s)} \tag{3.17}$$

where

$K_1 = 8.4034 \text{ min}$

$T_{c1} = 3.3484 \text{ min}$

$T_{c2} = 33.1663 \text{ min}$

$T_{c3} = 416.9103 \text{ min}$

$T_{c4} = 10 \text{ min}$

$T_{c5} = 18.1818 \text{ min}$

$T_{c6} = 303.0303 \text{ min}$

$\tau = 1/3 \text{ min}$

Table 3.2 Table representing the derived parameters of the Hill equation (3.18) for each of the 10 patients

Patient	Power α	$C_e(50)$ (μg ml^{-1})	E_{max} (mmHg)
1	4	1.03	−40
2	3	1.28	−50
3	4.5	1.36	−50
4	4	1.74	−55
5	4	1.50	−55
6	4	1.28	−25
7	4.5	1.32	−40
8	3.5	1.08	−45
9	4.5	1.42	−50
10	4	0.97	−30
Mean	4	1.3	−44
Standard deviation	0.45	0.22	−9.7

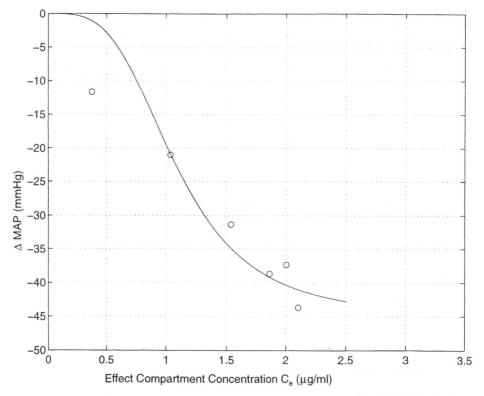

Figure 3.11 Curve fitting to propofol pharmacodynamics when $\alpha = 3.5$, $C_e = 1.08$ μg ml^{-1} and $E_{max} = -45$ mmHg.

3.4.5 Method for establishing the effect–concentration relationship

Most of the work hitherto conducted with respect to modelling propofol pharmacodynamics has utilised the EEG median frequency (Schuttler *et al.*, 1986; Schwilden *et al.*, 1989) or the awakening and orientation factors (Shafer *et al.*, 1988). These studies suggested a sigmoidal E_{max} model (Halford and Sheiner, 1981) between effect-compartment concentration and effect to form a nonlinear structure:

$$E = E_{max} \frac{C_e^\alpha}{C_e^\alpha + C_e(50)^\alpha} \tag{3.18}$$

Also, as far as mean arterial pressure is concerned, it is believed that such a sigmoidal relationship may be relevant since there exists, at clinical concentrations, a threshold below which no significant changes in mean arterial pressure are observed (see Section 3.1). Based on these facts, it was decided to fit a Hill equation to the effect relationship. In order to do that, the data Δ MAP against C_e for each patient were plotted, then the best fit was estimated and the approximate value of C_e (50) was determined. It should be noted that in all the plots the first point was ignored because it was likely to be erroneous since at that stage it is probable that the drug had not properly mixed with blood giving rise to an unrealistically high blood pressure value. A computer program was used to simulate equation (3.17) using a trial and error choice of the parameter α. Figure 3.11 is a sample plot from the ten studied plots for which satisfactory α and C_e (50) were achieved. Table 3.2 gives the values obtained for all of α and C_e (50) for each patient as well as their mean and SD quantities.

Hence, taking into account equation (3.17) and the combination of data from Table 3.2 and those derived from the later experiment, the nonlinear model describing the propofol model to changes in mean arterial blood pressure is obtained as that shown in Fig. 3.12.

3.5 A comparative control study using the propofol nonlinear model

It should be noted that our objective is to establish that if a control strategy uses a measured variable to realise feedback, then it is likely to lead to a better performance than any other form of control that only uses an average parameter model. This argument is reinforced more strongly when a large mismatch exists between the actual system parameters and those of the model. An intuitive explanation for this is that in the latter case since no output is actually measured, the controller is unable to make correction to its profile and carries on assuming that the model is correct. Hence, in order to enhance this argument the following experiments were performed in which matched and mismatch conditions between the patient parameters and those of the model were considered. Figure 3.13 is a schematic diagram representing the various blocks and variables involved when using both control strategies, i.e. GPC and modified Alvis algorithm.

3.5.1 Matched conditions

The first experiment consisted of using the modified Alvis algorithm with plasma concentration targets and observing the effect on MAP changes. In order to do that,

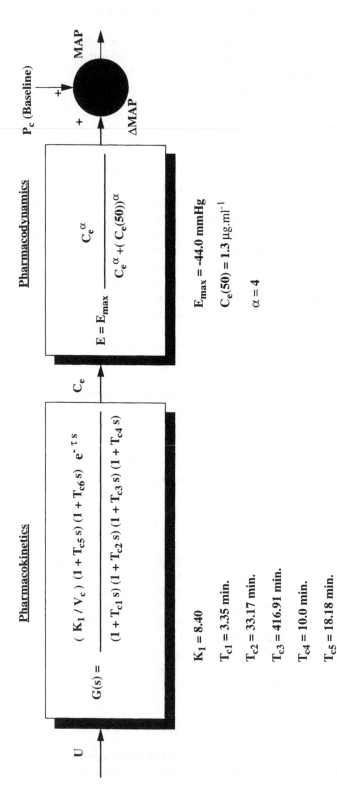

Figure 3.12 Diagram representing the overall nonlinear mean arterial pressure model associated with propofol.

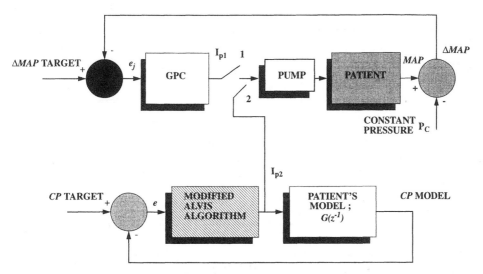

Figure 3.13 Schematic diagram representing the two types of control strategies associated with propofol infusion; either mode may be operated using the two software switches 1 and 2.

it is assumed here, and throughout, that *a priori* knowledge of the correspondence between plasma concentration and change in mean arterial pressure is known and is correct. Hence, using the Hill equation (equation (3.18)) in nominal conditions we found that a profile of -39 mmHg change in MAP for the 49 first samples, -20 mmHg from sample time 50 min to 99 min then back to -39 mmHg change corresponds to plasma concentrations of 2.17 μg ml^{-1}, 1.24 μg ml^{-1} then 2.17 μg ml^{-1} respectively. Using the latter target profile and assuming the same simulation conditions as in Section 3.3 with respect to the pharmacokinetics data, the sampling time, the high induction rate and the patient mass, the modified Alvis algorithm produced the performance of Figure 3.14 where it can be seen that the plasma concentration reached its target in a reasonable length of time during the three phases and the MAP reached its target more cautiously which is what anaesthetists favour.

Next, the fixed GPC algorithm was considered. A 1 minute sampling time (MAP readings from a Dinamap instrument are given at a minimum of 1 minute interval) was considered. The fixed GPC was allowed to run with a set of parameter estimates corresponding to the discrete model of equation (2.9) of 4 *a*s and 5 *b*s (the extra *b* parameter is for the fractional time delay) thought to reflect the best overall nonlinear structure. Moreover, the algorithm assumed a combination of (1, 10, 1, 0) for (N_1, N_2, NU, λ), a model following polynomial of $P(z^{-1}) = 10(1 - 0.9\ z^{-1})$ and an observer polynomial of $T(z^{-1}) = (1 - 0.85\ z^{-1})^2$. Set-point changes were known to the algorithm ten samples ahead. Figure 3.15 shows a good output performance together with a reasonably active control signal (clipped between 0 and 100 mg min^{-1}) whose effect on the plasma concentration can also be seen in the middle plot where a slight initial overshoot followed by an undershoot are apparent. These are due to the fact that the controlled variable in the GPC case is not CP but Δ MAP.

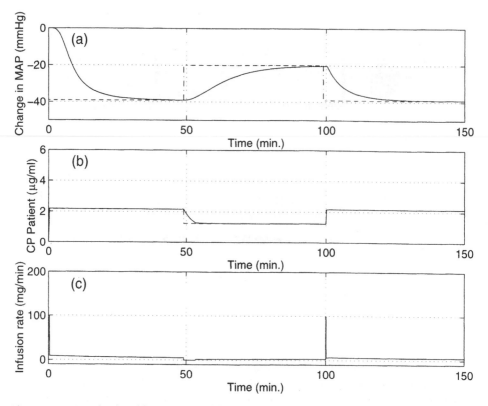

Figure 3.14   Pseudo closed-loop control of the nonlinear blood pressure model using the modified Alvis algorithm in the nominal case. (a) Solid line: patient's mean arterial pressure; dashdot line: target. (b) Patient's plasma concentration (CP). (c) Infusion rate profile.

3.5.2   Mismatch conditions

Using the standard deviation values published in Gepts *et al.* (1988), a mismatch between the patient's parameters and those of the model was considered. For the + 1 SD case, the modified Alvis algorithm, which uses nominal model parameters, led to the performance of Figure 3.16 which shows blood pressure and plasma concentration responses characterised by large offsets. However, the GPC algorithm, with the help of the filter polynomial $T(z^{-1})$, led to the performance of Figure 3.17 which shows good properties despite the fact that the controller had no knowledge about this mismatch and was hence operating assuming parameter estimates derived from the nominal model.

3.6   Conclusions

The study presented in this chapter completes a full circle in search of a control strategy which delivers the best possible infusion regimen for propofol during anaesthesia. Indeed, the investigation started by considering a protocol derived from early work by Alvis and co-workers (Alvis *et al.*, 1985) on fentanyl, later modified in Jannett (1986) and Maitre *et al.* (1986) and which usually leads to excellent regulation properties around target concentrations in both open- and closed-loop conditions,

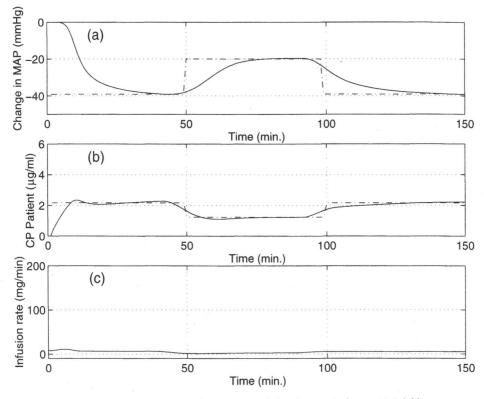

Figure 3.15 GPC of the nonlinear blood pressure model in the nominal case. (a) Solid line: patient's mean arterial pressure; dashdot line: target. (b) Patient's plasma concentration (CP). (c) Infusion rate profile.

providing that a relatively small sampling time is chosen (usually ≤ 10 seconds). It enables the controller to track closely the drug movement; although it is worth noting that it is not possible, in the case of this type of controller, to tailor the input signal as is possible with various other approaches. Our study which used this control strategy, mainly based on an average pharmacodynamic parameter population, showed that when a significant mismatch exists between the patient parameters and those of the model considered in the control law (as is usually the case), the performance degraded. The result is intuitively predictable since no real measurement is available for correction purposes. This result prompted the use of an alternative model-based controller, GPC, which would have the advantage, besides tailoring the response transient, of using a measurement signal and its variance to decide on the best input signal leading to a minimum value for its variance. The question of measurement which is crucial to the method is an open issue as far as anaesthesia is concerned, but suffice it to say here that early published work suggested that for certain drugs plasma concentrations are not the appropriate variables one should focus on (Schills *et al.*, 1987) but rather the effect they produce. This assertion is somewhat similar to the one which has been advanced recently by Jacobs and Williams (1993) in which it is argued that the concentration at the

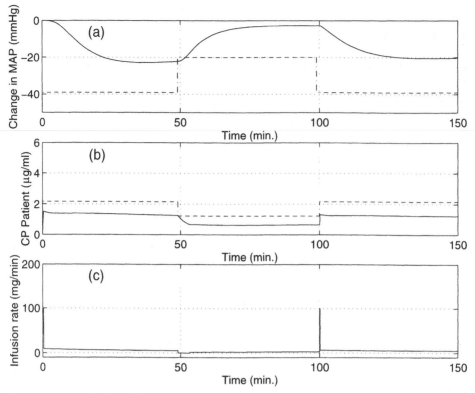

Figure 3.16 Psuedo closed-loop control of the nonlinear blood pressure model using the modified Alvis algorithm in the mismatch case. (a) Solid line: patient's mean arterial pressure; dashdot line: target. (b) Patient's plasma concentration (CP). (c) Infusion rate profile.

'effect compartment' is the proper variable to target. In light of these considerations, it was decided to perform a study that would model the direct effect associated with propofol. Analysis on data from ten patients revealed the existence of a hypothetical compartment linked to the central compartment by a rate constant equivalent to a half-life of 6.93 minutes. The next step consisted of establishing the relationship between the effect-compartment concentration and the produced effect itself. In order to do that one had to decide the nature of the effect upon which this relationship should be based. MAP was chosen as the effect variable for various reasons:

1. It represents an on-line quantifiable inferential indicator for depth of anaesthesia.

2. Reductions in blood pressure levels have been observed following propofol administration.

A Hill equation was fitted to the available data, completing, therefore, the blood pressure model associated with propofol, which is described by a fourth-order linear model followed by a strong nonlinearity represented by a Hill equation. Although some of the model parameters were identified using trial and error methods, it is believed that it represents a good approximation of the metabolism of the drug from the period it is administered intravenously to the patient. Simulation experiments

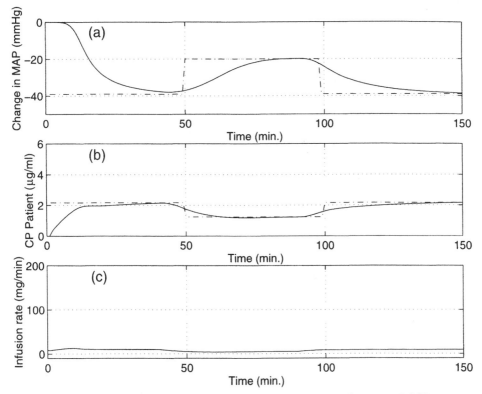

Figure 3.17   GPC of the nonlinear blood pressure model in the mismatch case. (a) Solid line: patient's mean arterial pressure; dashdot line: target. (b) Patient's plasma concentration (CP). (c) Infusion rate profile.

using the two algorithms previously cited, i.e. the modified Alvis algorithm and the GPC algorithm, showed that although under matched conditions their performances were comparable, GPC displays better robustness properties when a significant mismatch between the patient parameters and those of the model are present. This result reinforces the argument that GPC represents a real challenge to the type of control strategies devised by Alvis to control drug infusion, in this case propofol for induction of anaesthesia.

CHAPTER FOUR

Multivariable Generalised Predictive Control in the Operating Theatre

4.1 Introduction

Anaesthesia has been defined (see Chapter 1) as that part of the medical profession which ensures that the patient's body is insensitive to pain and possibly other stimuli during surgical operations and also after surgery. It includes muscle relaxation (paralysis), as described in Chapter 2, unconsciousness (state of sleep), and analgesia (pain relief). For muscle relaxation, we have already seen that measurements are made via evoked EMG responses obtained from supramaximal stimulation near the ulnar nerve at the elbow. Resulting EMG signals (electromyogram) at the hand are rectified and integrated, giving a proportional measurement of the degree of relaxation (i.e. induced paralysis). The drug used throughout this study is similar to the one previously considered, i.e. atracurium which is a modern, fast-acting agent suitable for continuous infusion via a motor-driven syringe pump.

In contrast, depth of anaesthesia is more difficult to quantify accurately. It is, in fact, agreed that there is no absolute standard for the clinical state of anaesthesia against which new methods designed to measure 'depth' of anaesthesia can be calibrated (Robb *et al.*, 1988). Thus, one approach has been to merge a number of clinical signs and on-line monitored data to produce an expert system advisor for the anaesthetist. This system, called RESAC, has been developed and validated in a series of clinical trials (Linkens *et al.*, 1990). In spite of the multi-sensor nature of the above approach, it appears that during the majority of operating periods when no unusual emergency conditions occur, a good indication of unconsciousness can be obtained from a single on-line monitored variable. Thus, the use of arterial blood pressure, monitored via an inflatable cuff using a Dinamap instrument, has been investigated for feedback control with simple PI strategies (Robb *et al.*, 1988). In this case the control actuation was via a stepper motor driving the dial on a gas vaporiser. This concept forms the basis for the modelling and control aspects of unconsciousness in the following work. In particular, we have used the drug isoflurane in these studies. This is an inhalational drug commonly used in modern surgery.

Section 4.2 describes the modelling approach used to derive the multivariable anaesthesia model, while Section 4.3 reviews the theoretical background behind multivariable GPC in its basic and extended forms. Section 4.4 presents a series of simulation experiments on the elicited multivariable model and Section 4.5 describes the multivariable control system which has been transferred to the operating theatre and the results of the clinical trials which were conducted on patients who underwent surgery normally requiring muscle relaxation as well as general anaesthesia. These trials are analysed and discussed in the same section. Finally, in Section 4.6 conclusions are drawn with respect to the practicality of the multivariable control system and the various benefits it offers the anaesthetist in the operating theatre.

4.2 Identification of the nonlinear anaesthesia model

The necessary transfer function components for the model used in these studies have been obtained in various ways. The two drugs considered in the model for human beings are atracurium (for producing muscle relaxation) and isoflurane (for inducing unconsciousness). The individual pathways are described in the following sections.

4.2.1 Atracurium mathematical model

Pharmacokinetics

The study conducted and reported in Chapter 2 gave the following equation:

$$\frac{X_1}{U_1} = \frac{9.94(1 + 10.64s)}{(1 + 3.08s)(1 + 34.42s)} \tag{4.1}$$

where X_1 and U_1 are the drug concentration in the blood and the drug input respectively.

Equation 4.1 describes the pharmacokinetics of the muscle relaxation system relating to the atracurium drug.

Pharmacodynamics

Similarly, to characterise the drug effect, the Hill equation is used to relate to a specific concentration giving the following expression:

$$E_{\text{eff}} = \frac{E_{\text{max}}}{1 + \dfrac{(0.404)^{2.98}}{(X_E)^{2.98}}} \tag{4.2}$$

where E_{eff}, E_{max} and X_E are the drug effect produced (paralysis), the maximum effect (paralysis) which can be produced, and the drug concentration in the effect compartment (see Chapter 2) respectively.

Finally, the overall transfer function describing the atracurium mathematical model is given by the following equation:

$$G_{11}(s) = \frac{X_E}{U_1} = \frac{K_1\, e^{-\tau_1 s}(1 + T_4 s)}{(1 + T_1 s)(1 + T_2 s)(1 + T_3 s)} \tag{4.3}$$

where

$$K_1 = 1.0$$

$$\tau_1 = 1 \text{ min}$$

$$T_1 = 4.81 \text{ min}$$

$$T_2 = 34.42 \text{ min}$$

$$T_3 = 3.08 \text{ min}$$

$$T_4 = 10.64 \text{ min}$$

4.2.2 Isoflurane unconsciousness model

Anaesthesia or unconsciousness is defined as being the state in which the body is insensitive to pain or other stimuli. There is no direct method of measuring depth of anaesthesia. Previous research work namely by Schwilden *et al.* (1987, 1989) and Savege *et al.* (1978) used quantitative EEG (electroencephalogram) analysis in humans to give an indication of their anaesthetic state. However, the interpretation of the tracings is a difficult and subjective task. The information proved unreliable even when interpreted by experienced staff, since the characteristic patterns are often disturbed by factors such as anoxia, surgical stimulations, and anaesthetic agents used (Breckenridge and Aitkenhead, 1983). Consequently, anaesthetists have to resort to the merger of several clinical signs such as blood pressure, respiration, etc. to obtain the closest possible indication of how well the patient is anaesthetised. Indeed, in a study conducted by Asbury (1990), anaesthetists were asked to rank the relative importance of ten clinical signs. These signs were ranked on a scale of 1 to 10 based on the mean values provided by these anaesthetists. Table 4.1 shows the result of this survey.

From these ten clinical signs, blood pressure has been selected as one variable to give indication of depth of anaesthesia. Gray and Asbury (1986) describe a system that controls systolic arterial pressure (SAP). The algorithm, a simple PI controller, achieved a quality of control ranging from good to fairly poor, and in most operations the patient recovered fairly quickly. It has been concluded from this study that when no emergency conditions occur, blood pressure could be used to provide a good indication of the patient's anaesthetic state. In fact, previous published work by Schills and co-workers (1987) used mean arterial pressure and a measure

Table 4.1 Anaesthetists' classification of the ten clinical signs by order of importance

Clinical sign	Mean of raw ranks	Order of mean rank
Movement and response to surgery	7.4	1
Respiration rate	5.8	2
Heart rate	5.3	3
Low muscle tone	5.0	4
Lacrimation	4.9	5
Arterial pressure	**4.84**	**6**
Sweating	4.77	7
Pupil position	4.6	8
Pupil diameter	3.4	9
Capillary refill	2.5	10

of EEG frequency to control anaesthesia via halothane in an on–off control strategy which was found to be less sensitive to parameter mismatches. It has also been argued that the lowest blood pressure that occurs normally during sleep is 15–20% less than the average pressure while awake. Elderly and hypotensive persons require a margin at 10%. Consequently, mean arterial pressure (MAP) is used as the second variable for the multivariable model considered throughout this study.

Off-line identification techniques such as maximum likelihood or instrumental variables methods should ideally be used to obtain an adequate and parsimonious discrete-time transfer function model of a locally linearised controllable system in adaptive control applications. Indeed, it is widely known from the literature that system identification has been possible in some biomedical applications, such as PRBS excitation of muscle relaxant drug response (Linkens *et al.*, 1982). However, it is not always possible to apply these methods within clinical environments, partly because of ethical considerations and also because of limitations in time. Anaesthetic drugs normally have stable and slow-acting responses, consequently, step and bolus responses are the most common identification procedures used by clinicians even though the signal-to-noise ratios are often very low. In light of the above considerations, a study was conducted by Millard *et al.* (1988a, 1988b), in which step response trials of several patients to isoflurane were carried out before and after self-tuning control of blood pressure during surgery. This was considered essential for safety reasons, because the authors used the early version of Clarke and Gawthrop's algorithm (1975) to control mean arterial blood pressure, and which was found to be sensitive to wrong time delay assumption. In a tranquil anaesthetised state, step responses to changes in inspired concentration of isoflurane from a vaporiser were performed. The patient's blood pressure response showed a transport delay. This pure dead-time is likely to vary slightly due to the breathing cycle of about 6 seconds. In fact, in the 55 patients studied, including 12 others in similar experiments conducted by the same author (Millard *et al.*, 1986), dead-times in the range 16–30 seconds have been observed. If the changes in inhaled isoflurane concentration are small (0–5%), then the responses can be approximated by linear characteristics. However, if the changes do not fall within this range, the responses are in general nonlinear and time varying.

Thus, a first-order linear model with dead-time has been adopted, having a time constant of 1–2 minutes. The magnitude of this time constant is large enough to absorb some inaccuracy of dead-time estimate due to breathing variations. On the other hand, in order to estimate the steady state gain, it is assumed that a relatively sensitive patient needs 2% isoflurane for a 30 mmHg reduction of the mean arterial pressure (Millard *et al.*, 1988b). Therefore, the model describing variation of blood pressure to small changes in inhaled isoflurane concentration can be written as:

$$G_{22}(s) = \frac{\Delta \text{ MAP}}{U_2} = \frac{K_2\, e^{-\tau_2 s}}{(1 + T_5\, s)} \tag{4.4}$$

where Δ MAP is the change in the arterial blood pressure and U_2 is the isoflurane drug input, and

$\tau_2 = 25$ seconds

$T_5 = 2$ min

$K_2 = -15$ mmHg/%

4.2.3 Interactive component model

Atracurium to mean arterial pressure (MAP) interaction

This interaction has been investigated in human beings and there seems to be small (clinically insignificant) changes in blood pressure. Most of these changes as a result of atracurium administration occur because it has a slight ability to release histamine. This is a very transient chemical effect in the blood lasting for no more than a minute and it does not appear in every patient (Asbury, 1990).

Isoflurane to muscle relaxation interaction

In order to identify this type of interaction which is small but significant, an experiment was performed by Asbury (1990), in which a patient, a man of 47 without a kidney but having a renal transplant, had to be anaesthetised. The following gives a description of the procedure adopted.

With the patient set-up and control readings of the Dinamap as well as of the Relaxograph taken, the patient was given a 10 mg dose of atracurium. This completely wiped out his EMG tracing (see Figure 4.1) which began to reappear 20 minutes later. An infusion of atracurium of 5 mg h^{-1} was then commenced. This continued for 50 minutes by which time a steady level had been achieved and this corresponding place on the trace is 1A in Figure 4.2 where a step-change in isoflurane concentration from 0–1% was introduced. At point 2A on the trace of Figure 4.3, the isoflurane was switched off. Now at this stage the experiment had already taken 1 hour and 35 minutes, at which time a new equilibrium was achieved. The isoflurane was again switched on to 1% at point 3A on the trace of Figure 4.4. Once the changes were observed, the isoflurane was finally switched off at point 4A on the trace of Figure 4.5. At point 5A on the trace of the same figure the effect of atracurium was reversed using a dose of neostigmine and glycopyrrolate with a satisfactory return to 100% baseline, suggesting that there had been very little drift.

In order to analyse this whole tracing, it is worth dividing the experiment into two main parts:

- The on-phases part (marks 1A and 3A).
- The off-phases part (marks 2A and 4A).

The point in proceeding in such a manner will become clearer in the forthcoming sections.

1. *The on-phases part* From Figure 4.2 where the EMG signal versus time is shown, it can be seen that after a 1% change of isoflurane has been introduced, the EMG signal started to decline following a time delay sequence of about 40 seconds. Moreover, if the isoflurane change is kept within a relatively small range (as in this very case), the shape of the transient clearly suggests a second-order linear model with a pure time delay of the form:

$$G_{1\,on}(s) = \frac{K_{on}\,e^{-\tau s}}{(1 + T_{1\,on}\,s)(1 + T_{2\,on}\,s)} \tag{4.5}$$

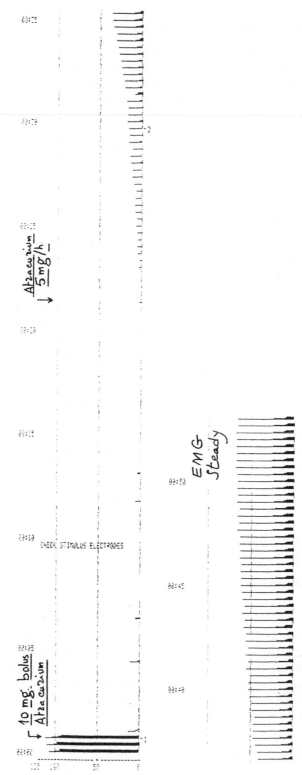

Figure 4.1 Recorded EMG corresponding to the first phase which follows the injection of the initial atracurium bolus dose.

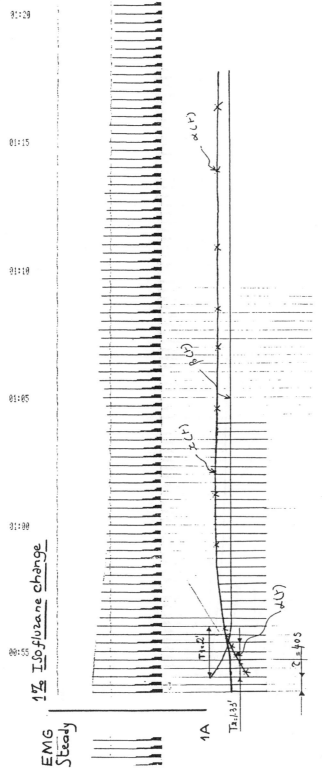

Figure 4.2 Recorded EMG corresponding to the phase which follows the introduction of a 1% isoflurane change at mark 1A.

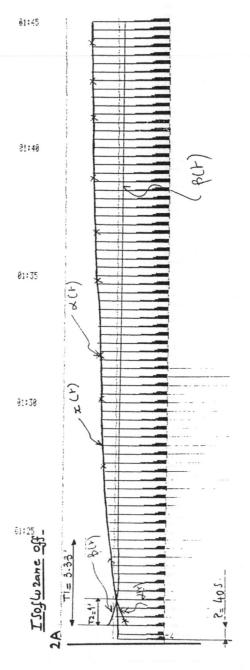

Figure 4.3 Recorded EMG when isoflurane was switched off at mark 2A.

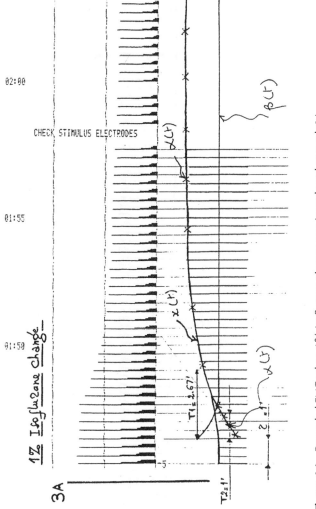

Figure 4.4 Recorded EMG when 1% isoflurane change was introduced at mark 3A.

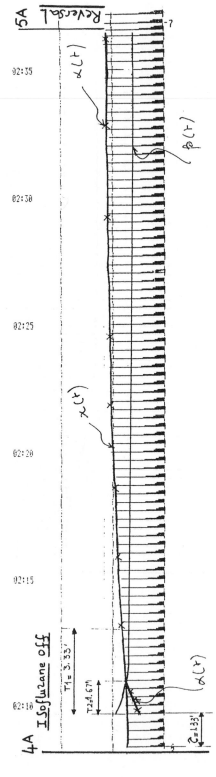

Figure 4.5 Recorded EMG when isoflurane was switched off at mark 4A and the blockade reversed at mark 5A.

Using the identification methods described in Graupe (1976), an attempt was made to evaluate the parameters in the above equation. It is, however, worth noting that for convenience the signal (100% − EMG) which is the paralysis was plotted. In order to evaluate the first time constant $T_{1\ \text{on}}$, it is assumed that for large t the curve referred to by $x(t)$ on the same figure is approximated by:

$$x(t) = x_\infty - x(t) = \text{coefficient}_1\ e^{-t/T_{1\text{on}}} = \alpha(t)$$

where $T_{1\ \text{on}}$ represents the dominant time constant.

Drawing the tangent at this curve referred to by $\alpha(t)$ gives:

$$T_{1\ \text{on}} \equiv 6 \text{ segments} \equiv 120 \text{ seconds} = 2 \text{ minutes}$$

If the curve given by the following equation is drawn, i.e.

$$\beta(t) = x(t) - \alpha(t) = \text{coefficient}_2\ e^{-t/T_{2\text{on}}}$$

where $T_{2\ \text{on}}$ is the smallest time constant, then drawing the tangent at the same curve leads to:

$$T_{2\ \text{on}} \equiv 4 \text{ segments} \equiv 80 \text{ seconds} = 1.33 \text{ minutes}$$

The final value theorem allows one to evaluate the steady state gain, i.e.:

$$x_\infty = 15\%$$

Therefore

$$K = 15\%/\% \text{ or } K = 0.15 \text{ (normalised input and output)}$$

Hence, the identified second-order model for this phase can be summarised by the following transfer function:

$$G_{1\ \text{on}}(s) = \frac{0.15\ e^{-0.67s}}{(1 + 2s)(1 + 1.33s)} \tag{4.6}$$

Following the same procedure as previously for the trace starting at point 3A on Figure 4.4, the following transfer function was obtained:

$$G_{2\ \text{on}}(s) = \frac{0.33\ e^{-s}}{(1 + 2.67s)(1 + s)} \tag{4.7}$$

Taking the mean values for the two transfer functions yields:

$$G_{\text{on}}(s) = \frac{0.24\ e^{-0.84s}}{(1 + 2.33s)(1 + 1.17s)} \tag{4.8}$$

2. *The off-phases part* The point in analysing these parts of the transient where the isoflurane was switched off after a certain equilibrium has been reached, is mainly to establish the *symmetry* of a possible linear model reinforcing, hence its validity, and justifying the assumption of the model being linear for small changes of input.

In light of these considerations, the same procedure of section 1 above was conducted using Figures 4.3 and 4.5, leading to the following results:

$$G_{1\ \text{off}}(s) = \frac{0.31\ e^{-0.67s}}{(1 + 3.33s)(1 + s)} \tag{4.9}$$

$$G_{2\ \text{off}}(s) = \frac{0.28\ e^{-1.33s}}{(1 + 3.33s)(1 + 1.67s)} \tag{4.10}$$

Taking the mean values for the two transfer functions 4.9 and 4.10 yields:

$$G_{off}(s) = \frac{0.29 \, e^{-s}}{(1 + 3.33s)(1 + 1.33s)} \tag{4.11}$$

A quick analysis of these two transfer functions did indeed suggest that the model is more or less symmetrical considering the fact that the study has been performed entirely by manual means.

Hence, if an overall model describing the effect that isoflurane has on muscle relaxation is required, mean values should be taken between the two models, thus giving:

$$G_{12}(s) = \frac{K_4 \, e^{-\tau_3 s}}{(1 + T_6 s)(1 + T_7 s)} \tag{4.12}$$

where

$$K_4 = 0.27\%/\%$$

$$\tau_3 = 1 \text{ min}$$

$$T_6 = 1.25 \text{ min}$$

$$T_7 = 2.83 \text{ min}$$

Equation 4.12 represents the final linear transfer function which describes the effect of the inhaled agent isoflurane on muscle relaxation during surgery.

4.2.4   Overall multivariable anaesthetic model

In light of the above identification studies, the overall linear multivariable system combining muscle relaxation together with anaesthesia (in terms of mean arterial blood pressure measurements), whose components are also illustrated in Figure 4.6, can be summarised by the following equation:

$$\begin{bmatrix} \text{Paralysis} \\ \Delta \text{ MAP} \end{bmatrix} = \begin{bmatrix} G_{11}(s) & G_{12}(s) \\ 0 & G_{22}(s) \end{bmatrix} \begin{bmatrix} U_1 \\ U_2 \end{bmatrix} \tag{4.13}$$

where

$$G_{11}(s) = \frac{1.0 \, e^{-s}(1 + 10.64s)}{(1 + 3.08s)(1 + 4.81s)(1 + 34.42s)}$$

$$G_{12}(s) = \frac{0.27 \, e^{-s}}{(1 + 2.83s)(1 + 1.25s)} \tag{4.14}$$

$$G_{22}(s) = \frac{-15.0 \, e^{-0.42s}}{(1 + 2s)}$$

Finally, the overall nonlinear multivariable system combining all the effects is obtained by including the nonlinearity described previously contained in the muscle relaxation path.

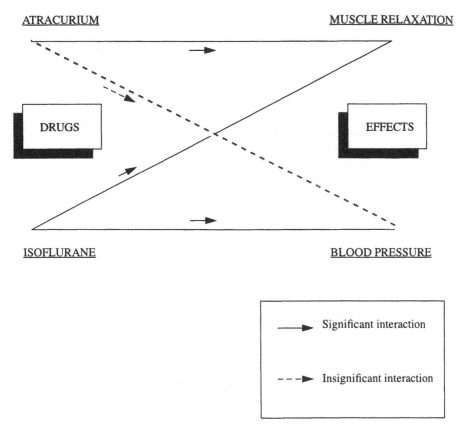

ATRACURIUM   MUSCLE RELAXATION

DRUGS   EFFECTS

ISOFLURANE   BLOOD PRESSURE

| | Significant interaction |
| | Insignificant interaction |

Figure 4.6 Schematic diagram representing the different components forming the multivariable anaesthetic model.

4.3 Development of the multivariable GPC algorithm for anaesthesia

4.3.1 The basic algorithm

Consider the m-input m-output linear discrete-time system:

$$A(z^{-1})y(t) = z^{-k_{ij}}B(z^{-1})u(t-1) + \frac{C(z^{-1})\xi(t)}{\Delta} \tag{4.15}$$

where

$$A(z^{-1}) = I + A_1 z^{-1} + A_2 z^{-2} + \ldots + A_n z^{-n}$$

$$B(z^{-1}) = B_1 + B_2 z^{-1} + B_3 z^{-2} + \ldots + B_m z^{-m+1}$$

$$C(z^{-1}) = C_0 + C_1 z^{-1} + C_2 z^{-2} + \ldots + C_p z^{-p}$$

$$y(t) = [y_1(t), y_2(t), \ldots, y_m(t)]$$

$$u(t) = [u_1(t), u_2(t), \ldots, u_m(t)]$$

$$\Delta = 1 - z^{-1}$$

$y(t)$ and $u(t)$ are vectors of m measurable outputs and m measurable inputs respectively; k_{ij} is the integral time delay of the ijth element of $B(z^{-1})$, and $\xi(t)$ denotes a vector of m uncorrelated sequences of random variables with zero mean and covariance σ.

In order to derive a j-step ahead predictor of $y(t + j)$ based on equation (4.15), assume that $C(z^{-1}) = I$ with no loss of generality and consider the following Diophantine equation:

$$I = E_j A(z^{-1})\Delta + z^{-j}F_j(z^{-1}) \tag{4.16}$$

where E_j and F_j are matrix polynomials defined given the matrix polynomial $A(z^{-1})$ and the prediction interval j. Following the same procedure as in the SISO case of Chapter 2, it can be shown that the predictor becomes:

$$\begin{aligned} \hat{y}(t + j) &= G_j \Delta u(t + j - 1) + F_j(z^{-1})y(t) \\ G_j &= E_j(z^{-1})B(z^{-1}) \end{aligned} \tag{4.17}$$

Equation (4.17) can be rewritten as follows:

$$\left[\begin{aligned} \hat{y}(t + 1) &= G_1 \Delta u(t) + F_1 Y(t) \\ \hat{y}(t + 2) &= G_2 \Delta u(t + 1) + F_2 y(t) \\ &\vdots \qquad\qquad \vdots \qquad\qquad \vdots \\ \hat{y}(t + N) &= G_N \Delta u(t + N - 1) + F_N y(t) \end{aligned} \right. \tag{4.18}$$

Consider now a cost function of the following form:

$$\left[\begin{aligned} J_{GPC} &= E[(Q1 + Q2)] \\ Q1 &= \sum_{j=N_1}^{N_2} [y(t + j) - \omega(t + j)]^T [y(t + j) - \omega(t + j)] \\ Q2 &= \sum_{j=1}^{N_2} [\Delta u(t + j - 1)^T \Lambda(j) \Delta u(t + j - 1)] \end{aligned} \right. \tag{4.19}$$

with the variables and indices bearing the same definitions as in Chapter 2, except that $\Lambda(j)$ is the control weighting sequence and is a diagonal matrix.

Since only the first increment is considered, the solution for the minimisation of the previous cost can be summarised as the following:

$$\tilde{u} = (G^T G + \Lambda I)^{-1}G^T(\omega - f)$$

f denoting signals in equation (4.18) which are known at time t, or:

$$\Delta u(t) = (I_m, 0, 0, \ldots, 0)(G^T G + \Lambda I)^{-1}G^T(\omega - f) \tag{4.20}$$

where

$$G = \begin{bmatrix} H_0 & 0 & \ldots & 0 \\ H_1 & H_0 & \ldots & \\ H_2 & H_1 & \ldots & \\ H_3 & H_2 & \ldots & \\ \vdots & \vdots & & \vdots \\ H_{N2-1} & H_{N2-2} & \ldots & H_0 \end{bmatrix}$$

$H_0, \ldots, H_{N2-1}$ are submatrices of dimension $m \times m$, m being the number of channels within the matrix G which itself is of dimension $(m \times N_2)(m \times N_2)$ (Mohtadi, 1986).

As in the SISO case, the GPC approach uses the powerful assumption that after a certain horizon NU all control increments are equal to zero, which reduces considerably the computational burden since the matrix G becomes:

$$
\bar{G} = \begin{bmatrix}
H_0 & 0 & \cdots & 0 \\
H_1 & H_0 & \cdots & \\
H_2 & H_1 & \cdots & \\
H_3 & H_2 & \cdots & \\
\vdots & \vdots & & \vdots \\
H_{N2-1} & H_{N2-2} & \cdots & H_{N2-NU}
\end{bmatrix}
$$

The above development ignores the fact that the output costing horizons N_{2m} and the control costing horizons NU_m could be different for the m different channels. If, however, the user judges them to be different, some modifications have to be made to the algorithm, thus adding more flexibility and robustness to the design, especially if the process dealt with reflects a large difference in the dynamics from one channel to another. If the m channels have different output costing horizons $N_2(\text{ch } 1)$, $N_2(\text{ch } 2)$, ..., then every channel would have its rows in the $\bar{G}$ matrix equal to *zero* values from its own horizon $+1$ to the greatest horizon. If, however, the m channels have different control horizons, $NU(\text{ch } 1)$, $NU(\text{ch } 2)$, ..., then all the columns in the matrix $\bar{G}$ corresponding to the associated control increments would be made equal to *zero* and taken out of the matrix to avoid singularity.

Finally for fine tuning, Λ, the control weighting sequence, can be used to reduce control activity and improve robustness. A suitable form for Λ is:

$$\Lambda = \lambda \Sigma G^T G$$

where λ can take values between 0.0 and 1.0. If a value of 1.0 is used, for instance, then the term $(G^T \cdot G + \Lambda)^{-1}$ would have $1/2$ as a multiplicative coefficient, thus halving the control activity.

4.3.2 Inclusion of the model-following polynomial $P(z^{-1})$

For this purpose, let us consider the auxiliary output $\Psi(t)$ such that:

$$\Psi(t) = P(z^{-1})y(t)$$

$$P(z^{-1}) = P_N(z^{-1})(P_D(z^{-1}))^{-1} \tag{4.21}$$

The controller therefore minimises the following cost function which is, in fact, the expectation subject to data available at time t:

$$J(N_1, N_2) = \sum_{j=N_1}^{N_2} [\Psi(t+j) - \omega(t+j)]^2 + \sum_{j=1}^{N_2} \Lambda(j)(\Delta u(t+j-1))^2 \tag{4.22}$$

In this case the following Diophantine equation is considered:

$$P_N(z^{-1})(P_D(z))^{-1} = E_j A(z^{-1})\Delta + z^{-j}F_j(P_D(z^{-1}))^{-1} \qquad j = 1, 2, \ldots \tag{4.23}$$

It can be shown that this reduces to the following system of two equations:

$$\begin{cases} \Psi(t+j) = G_j(z^{-1})\Delta u(t+j-1) + F_j(z^{-1})(P_D(z^{-1}))^{-1}y(t) \\ G_j(z^{-1}) = E_j(z^{-1})B(z^{-1}) \end{cases} \qquad (4.24)$$

Following the same procedure as in the previous section the operation of minimisation results in the projected control increment vector with the form:

$$\begin{cases} \tilde{u} = (G^T G + \Delta I)^{-1} G^T(\omega - ff) \\ u(t) = u(t-1) + g^T(\omega - ff) \end{cases} \qquad (4.25)$$

where ff denotes signals in equation (4.24) known at time t, and g^T comprises the m rows of the matrix $(G^T G + \Lambda I)^{-1} G^T$.

Finally, it is worth noting at this stage that, as in the SISO case and in process control, $P(z^{-1})$ could be interpreted as being a model-reference polynomial which could penalise the overshoot, or reject a disturbance. It is particularly helpful when the value of NU is greater than 1 which causes the control signal to be highly active. The use of $P(z^{-1})$ affects both the set-point response as well as the disturbance rejection properties of the process under consideration.

4.3.3 Inclusion of the observer polynomial $T(z^{-1})$

Following the same procedure adopted in the previous sections, consider the following Diophantine equation:

$$T(z^{-1}) = E_j A\Delta + z^{-j}F_j \qquad (4.26)$$

where $T(z^{-1})$ is defined as a polynomial in the backward shift z^{-1} of degree 's' and of the form:

$$T(z^{-1}) = I + T_1 z^{-1} + T_2 z^{-2} + \ldots + T_s z^{-s}$$

The resulting prediction equations can be summarised as follows:

$$y(t+j) = T^{-1}[G_j \Delta u(t+j-1) + F_j y(t)] + T^{-1}E_j x(t+j)$$
$$G_j = E_j B \qquad (4.27)$$

For the controller to be optimal, the residual $T^{-1} E_j x(t+j)$ must be orthogonal to data at time t, suggesting that T and $x(t+j)$ are uncorrelated which is not always the case, leading therefore, to sub-optimal predictions. However, the choice of T as diagonal and with identical elements in each row implies commutativity of the product of matrices in equation (4.27) reducing considerably the computational burden. The following set of prediction equations is finally obtained:

$$y(t+j) = G_j \Delta u^f(t+j-1) + F_j y^f(t)$$
$$y^f(t) = T^{-1}y(t) \qquad (4.28)$$
$$u^f(t) = T^{-1}u(t)$$

Because the minimisation of the cost function is in terms of Δu and not Δu^f, the following equation is considered:

$$G_j = G'_j T + z^{-j}\Gamma_j \qquad (4.29)$$

where the coefficients of G'_j are equivalent to those of G_j when $T(z^{-1}) = I$. Consequently, equation (4.28) can be rewritten as:

$$y(t + j) = G'_j \Delta u(t + j - 1) + z^{-j} \Gamma \Delta u^f(t + j - 1) + F_j y^f(t) \qquad (4.30)$$

The minimisation procedure follows the same steps as in the previous sections.

Note that the modelling of multivariable system dynamics is usually expressed in terms of a set of ordinary differential equations which can be translated into the state-space form, details of which are given in Appendix I.

4.4 Simulation results

4.4.1 Simulation experiments using nominal parameter values

Several studies have involved the simulation of the model described in Section 4.2 using a fourth-order Runge–Kutta method with a fixed step integration interval of 0.1 and a sampling interval of 1 minute. Command signals of 80% then 70% for relaxation, and 80 mmHg then 70 mmHg for blood pressure were assumed throughout. Initial conditions were 0% relaxation and 100 mmHg mean arterial pressure. During the first 25 samples, initial control was provided by the self-tuner itself but with fixed parameter estimates obtained from the nominal linear model. The input signal was clipped between 0 and 1.0 for the atracurium drug input, and between 0% and 5% for the isoflurane input. For parameter estimation a UDU factorisation method (Bierman, 1977) was used on incremental data, with an initial covariance matrix and forgetting factor given by $Cov = 10^2.I$ and $\rho = 0.995$, respectively. A discrete multivariable model of 5 diagonal A matrices and 5 upper triangular B matrices (Wittenmark et al., 1987) of the form given below was estimated with an assumed time delay of 1 sample:

$$B(z^{-1}) = \begin{bmatrix} b_{11} & b_{12} \\ 0 & b_{22} \end{bmatrix} + \begin{bmatrix} b_{13} z^{-1} & b_{14} z^{-1} \\ 0 & b_{24} z^{-1} \end{bmatrix} + \cdots + \begin{bmatrix} b_{1(2m+1)} z^{-m} & b_{1(2m+2)} z^{-m} \\ 0 & b_{2(2m+2)} z^{-m} \end{bmatrix}$$

and

$$A(z^{-1}) = I + \begin{bmatrix} a_{13} z^{-1} & 0 \\ 0 & a_{24} z^{-1} \end{bmatrix} + \begin{bmatrix} a_{15} z^{-2} & 0 \\ 0 & a_{26} z^{-2} \end{bmatrix} + \cdots$$
$$+ \begin{bmatrix} a_{1(2n+1)} z^{-n} & 0 \\ 0 & a_{2(2n+2)} z^{-n} \end{bmatrix}$$

The experiments were conducted in 6 phases. Phases 1 to 4 used the basic algorithm, in contrast to phases 5 and 6 which were concerned with the extended algorithm using respectively the model following $P(z^{-1})$ and the observer polynomial $T(z^{-1})$. Figure 4.7 illustrates the configuration of the overall multivariable anaesthesia control system.

Figure 4.8 shows a result from phase 1 where the controller parameter settings were $(1, 10, 1, 0)$ for (N_1, N_2, NU, λ). This experiment gave well-damped responses

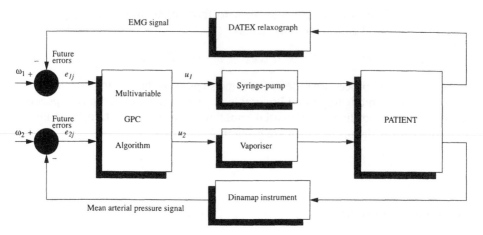

Figure 4.7 Diagram representing the multivariable anaesthesia control system associated with GPC.

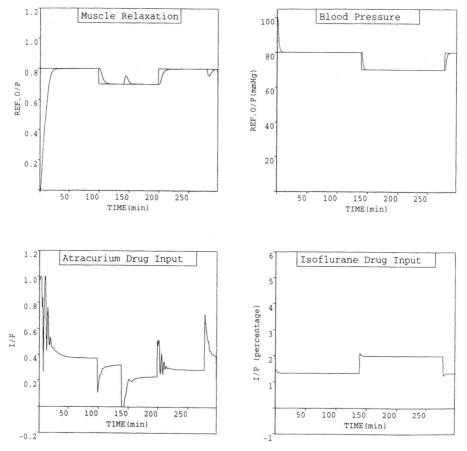

Figure 4.8 Closed-loop responses of the multivariable anaesthetic model under basic multivariable GPC with $N_1 = 1$; $N_2 = 10$; $NU = 1$.

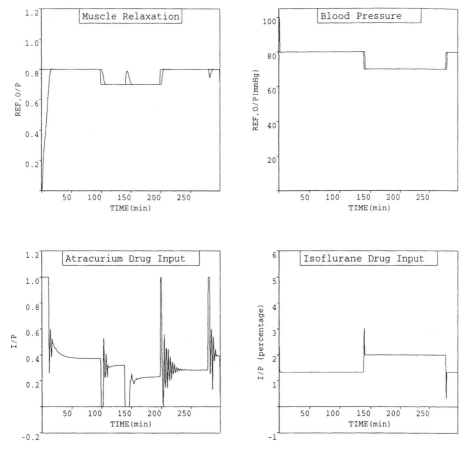

Figure 4.9 Closed-loop responses of the multivariable anaesthetic model under basic multivariable GPC with $N_1 = 1$; $N_2 = 10$; $NU = 2$.

for both channels but with some levels of interaction in the muscle relaxation channel. Phase 2 was concerned with the control horizon parameter NU which is considered to represent the corner-stone of the GPC algorithm (Clarke *et al.*, 1987a). In this experiment, its value was taken to be 2 and produced the response of Figure 4.9, where the transients in both channels were very fast. However, the response in the relaxation channel displayed a high level of interaction at time 140 minutes with a relatively active control signal thereafter. This was to be expected, since a value of $NU \geq 2$ always causes high control activity. Phase 3 shows how the controller parameter settings can be chosen to be different between the two channels: $N_1 = 1$, $N_2(\text{ch } 1) = 10$, $N_2(\text{ch } 2) = 20$, $NU(\text{ch } 1) = 1$, $NU(\text{ch } 2) = 2$. The result shown in Figure 4.10 also gave well-damped responses in both channels but with a high level of interaction due to the output horizon in the blood pressure channel which was 20 and this has the effect of increasing the level of channel-to-channel decoupling (Mohtadi, 1986). Figure 4.11 shows how the high control activity induced by a large control horizon NU can be reduced by the use of a non-zero

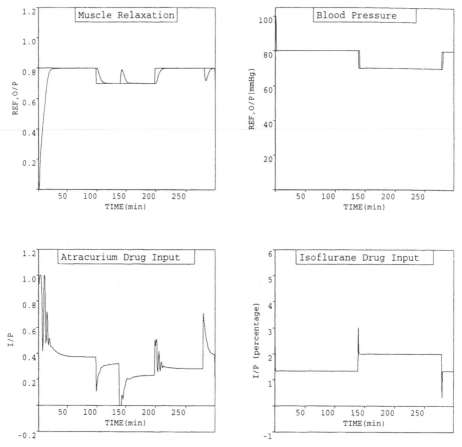

Figure 4.10   Investigation of differential channel parameters; $N_1 = 1$; N_2(ch 1) = 10; N_2(ch 2) = 20; NU(ch 1) = 1; NU(ch 2) = 2.

control weighting sequence λ ($\lambda = 1.0$), but on the other hand this has the effect of increasing the level of interactions between channels as seen here in the muscle relaxation channel. Another alternative which can be utilised in order to reduce channel-to-channel interactions is the use of the important model-following polynomial $P(z^{-1})$ which has the advantage of reducing the system's closed-loop bandwidth, and hence reducing the middle frequency decoupling. Based on the system's dynamics as well as the sampling period, a value of the polynomial time constant $T_c = 9.49$ minutes (identical for both channels) was selected for assignment of the $P(z^{-1})$ matrix. Figure 4.12 shows how this can be used to reduce the previous overshoot in relaxation as well as minimising the interaction, at the cost of over damping for the arterial pressure. Finally, Phase 6 considered the inclusion of the observer polynomial $T(z^{-1})$ together with the previous polynomial $P(z^{-1})$ in order to enhance further the robustness of the whole control strategy (Robinson and Clarke, 1991). Figure 4.13 shows how the effect of disturbances of 6% and 7 mmHg in the muscle relaxation channel and the blood pressure channel respectively can be

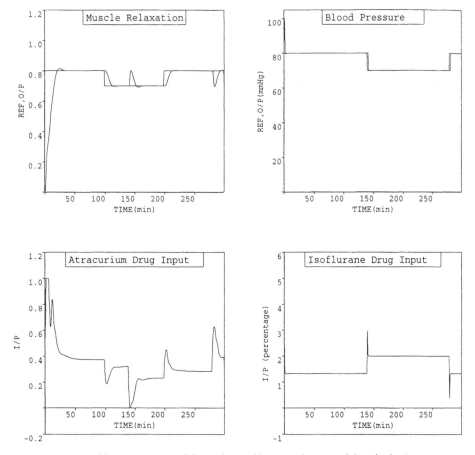

Figure 4.11 Closed-loop responses of the multivariable anaesthetic model under basic multivariable GPC with $N_1 = 1$; $N_2 = 10$; $NU = 2$; $\lambda = 1.0$.

reduced with the use of the $T(z^{-1})$ polynomial and at the same time modify the overall closed-loop responses with the use of the $P(z^{-1})$ polynomial.

4.4.2 Simulation experiments using bolus doses

In this part of the simulation study, experiments which mimic the actions of the anaesthetist in the operating theatre are conducted, in which bolus doses of atracurium are first administered to the patient to induce rapid paralysis (see Chapter 2). The same simulation conditions as above were considered except that a bolus dose of atracurium of 67 mg at 1 mg ml^{-1} concentration was initially applied for one sample to input u_1 and input u_2 was kept at 0. While the bolus effect took place, the loop remained open until the output in the muscle relaxation channel reached the safety level of 85%, at which point the loop was closed. The self-tuner was allowed to run with the initial parameter estimates until sample time 39 min (where a steady

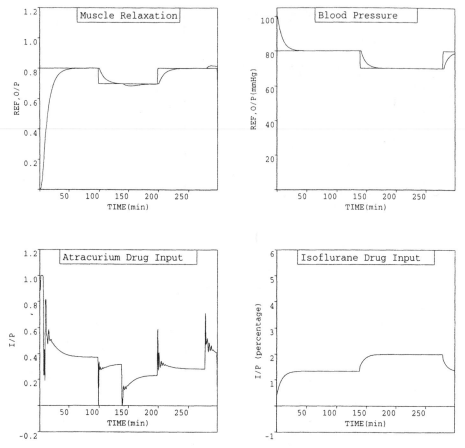

Figure 4.12 Extended multivariable GPC algorithm with model-following polynomial $P(z^{-1})$: $N_1 = 1$; $NU = 2$; $P = 10(1 - 0.9\ z^{-1}).I.$

state can be considered to have been safely reached) at which time the parameter estimation routine was allowed to be operational. The multivariable GPC algorithm was assigned the following tuning parameters:

$$N_1 = 1; \quad N_2 = 10; \quad NU(\text{ch 1}) = 2; \quad NU(\text{ch 2}) = 1;$$

$$P = \begin{bmatrix} \dfrac{(1 - 0.7z^{-1})}{0.3} & 0 \\ 0 & \dfrac{(1 - 0.9z^{-1})}{0.1} \end{bmatrix}$$

and $T(z^{-1}) = (1 - 0.8z^{-1})^2.I$ for control and estimation.

Figure 4.14 shows the result of the experiment where it can be seen that both outputs behaved very well with the interaction in the muscle relaxation channel reduced to a very low level. The blood pressure signal may seem slightly over-damped with a sluggish control signal, but this is very much favoured by anaes-thetists since it represents a cautious approach to the set-point without the risk of

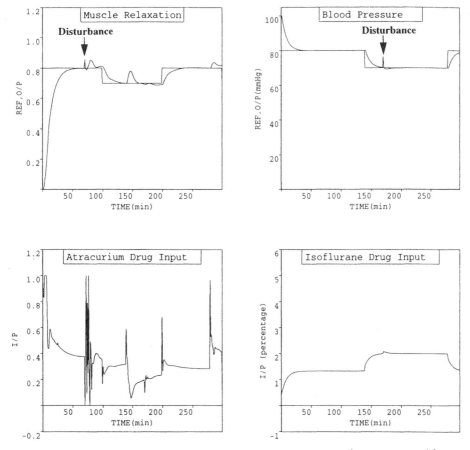

Figure 4.13 Effect of output disturbances with observed polynomial $T(z^{-1}) = (1 - 0 \, 8 \, z^{-1})^2 . I$ and model-following polynomial $P(z^{-1}) = 10(1 - 0.9 \, z^{-1})^2 . I$; $N_2 = 10$; $NU = 2$.

overshoot. When noise sequences of 1% and 5 mmHg were superimposed on the paralysis and blood pressure outputs respectively, the experiment produced the output responses of Figure 4.15 where the filter seems to have dealt effectively with the noise in both channels, especially in the muscle relaxation channel where a high control horizon of $NU = 2$ was chosen. It can also be noticed that the interactions in the muscle relaxation channel were at very low levels.

4.5 Clinical evaluation of the multivariable anaesthesia control system

The multivariable anaesthesia control system used in the operating theatre is illustrated in Figure 4.16 and consists of the following components:

- A Datex Relaxograph system for measuring the degree of muscle relaxation (paralysis).

- A Braun Perfusor Secura digital pump driving a disposable 50 ml/60 ml syringe containing a solution of atracurium calibrated between a minimum of 0 ml h^{-1} to a maximum of 99.99 ml h^{-1}.

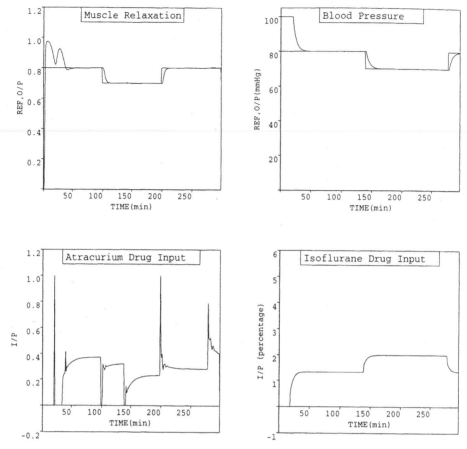

Figure 4.14 Effect of bolus doses in the noise-free case: $T(z^{-1}) = (1 - 0.8\,z^{-1})^2.I;$

$$P(z^{-1}) = \begin{bmatrix} \dfrac{(1 - 0.7z^{-1})}{0.3} & 0 \\ 0 & \dfrac{(1 - 0.9z^{-1})}{0.1} \end{bmatrix}$$

- A Datascope-3000 instrument which provides systolic arterial pressure (SAP) measurements every minute.

- An Enfluratec 3 vaporiser (Cyprane), for delivering isoflurane, modified to allow it to be driven by a stepper motor under computer control and calibrated between a minimum of 0% and a maximum of 5% with increments of 0.5%. The system for controlling the vaporiser contained various features which guarantee its safe use (Robb *et al.*, 1988).

- An IBM-compatible microcomputer which incorporates the control algorithm.

The links between the Datex Relaxograph, the Datascope-3000, and the Perfusor-Secura pump were via three RS-232 serial ports, whereas the communication with the vaporiser was via the parallel port.

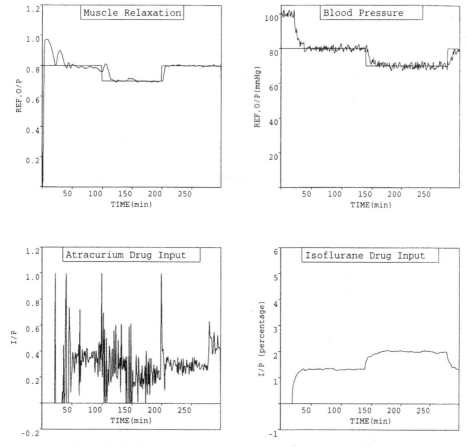

Figure 4.15 Effect of bolus doses in the stochastic case: $T(z^{-1}) = (1-0.8\ z^{-1})^2.I$;

$$P(z^{-1}) = \begin{bmatrix} \dfrac{(1 - 0.7z^{-1})}{0.3} & 0 \\ 0 & \dfrac{(1 - 0.9z^{-1})}{0.1} \end{bmatrix}$$

It is worth noting that in this series of clinical trials, systolic arterial pressure (SAP) rather than mean arterial pressure (MAP) signals were used as measurements.

4.5.1 Clinical preparation of the patients before surgery

Similarly to the trials conducted with the SISO version of GPC, in these trials the patients were selected with the knowledge that they did not suffer from a typical sensitivity to anaesthetic drugs because of myoneural disorders. They all underwent abdominal and keyhole surgery which normally requires muscle relaxation as well as general anaesthesia. Well before surgery (approximately 1 hour), a very fast acting muscle relaxant called suxamethonium was administered to enable the introduction of breathing tubes, and the trachea was intubated when the EMG reached a 15% value. The lungs were inflated with 30% oxygen and 70% nitrous oxide. While

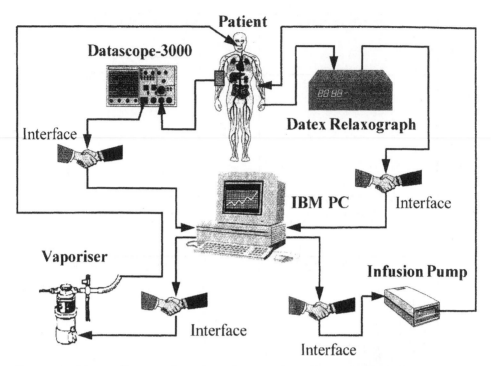

Figure 4.16   Diagram illustrating the multivariable control system set-up in the operating theatre.

still in the anaesthetic room, doses of morphine were administered, and the Relaxo-graph electrodes were placed on the patient's arm, and the calibration proceeded. The Datascope inflatable cuff was also placed on the other arm in order to record the baseline arterial pressure before any isoflurane administration. Once transferred to the theatre, the patient, who was now connected to the control system of Figure 4.16, was intravenously given an initial bolus dose of atracurium varying between 8 and 15 mg with a concentration of 1000 μg ml^{-1}.

4.5.2   Results and discussions

After local Ethics Committee approval, three patients were selected for the experi-ments as they all underwent surgery which requires muscle relaxation as well as general anaesthesia. The automatically controlled infusion of atracurium and administration of isoflurane (closed-loop mode) was started when T_1 reached a value of 10–15% of the 100% baseline value. Once the closed-loop mode was entered, a fixed controller in the shape of multivariable GPC with frozen parameter estimates, derived from average population dynamics, was established for 29 minutes after which adaptation was switched on. EMG measurements were taken every 20 seconds and three data measurements were averaged over a 1 minute inter-val with a 20% EMG target, whereas blood pressure measurements were taken at 1 minute intervals with the target being taken as a drop of 10% from the baseline systolic pressure (SAP) measured prior to surgery (baseline). For parameter estima-tion a UDU-factorisation method was used on incremental data with initial covari-

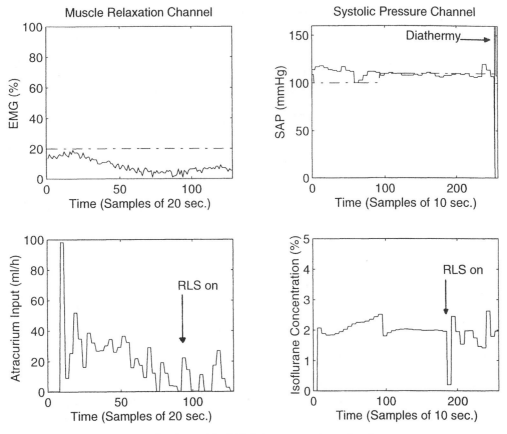

Figure 4.17 Performance of multivariable GPC during surgery for patient 1.

ance matrix and forgetting factor given by: $Cov = 10.I$ and $\rho = 0.999$, respectively. As in Section 4.4, a multivariable P-canonical model of 5 diagonal $A(z^{-1})$ matrices together with 5 upper triangular $B(z^{-1})$ matrices was used. It is worth noting that for the muscle relaxation channel EMG readings were obtained and updated every 20 seconds and averaged over three samples to get one EMG value over 1 minute, whereas the *same* SAP readings were transmitted through the RS-232 port every 10 seconds but *updated* every 1 minute. Hence, in the following data plots, the time axis in the muscle relaxation channel will be sub-divided in samples of 20 seconds, whereas the time axis in the SAP channel will be sub-divided in samples of 10 seconds.

Patient 1

For this trial the GPC controller had the following parameters:

$$N_1 = 1; \quad N_2 = 10; \quad NU(\text{ch 1}) = 1; \quad NU(\text{ch 2}) = 1$$

$$\lambda = 0; \quad P = \begin{bmatrix} \dfrac{(1 - 0.9z^{-1})}{0.1} & 0 \\ 0 & 1 \end{bmatrix}$$

$T(z^{-1}) = (1 - 0.8z^{-1})^2 I$ for control and estimation

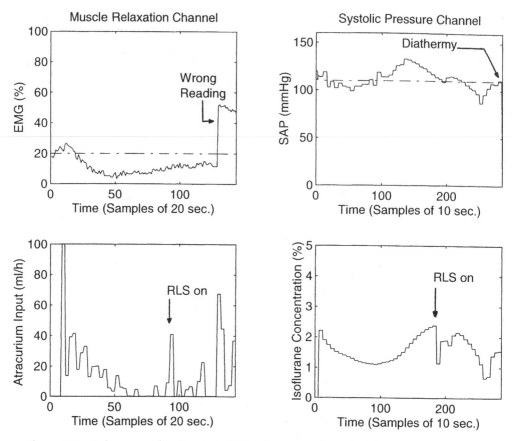

Figure 4.18   Performance of multivariable GPC during surgery for patient 2.

The idea behind the choice of a slow $P(z^{-1})$ pole was to force the EMG signal to track the target cautiously without inducing an undershoot which is undesirable in muscle relaxation management. Figure 4.17 shows the GPC performance under these conditions. The top plots correspond to the system's outputs whereas the bottom ones are for the system's inputs. As the figure shows the muscle relaxant channel was rather slow to converge to the target due to the choice of $P(z^{-1})$, whereas the systolic pressure channel shows that, despite an isoflurane input of about 2%, the SAP would not converge to the 100 mmHg target; this is believed to be due to the fact that at that time the surgeon was in the process of cutting tissues which made the blood pressure jump to almost 120 mmHg for about 16 minutes at which time the anaesthetist decided that a 110 mmHg target was more appropriate. This made the output track the target very efficiently with minimum activity even when the adaptation was turned on. The whole operation lasted 40 minutes after which the surgeon ordered the administration of both drugs to be ceased.

Patient 2

Using the same controller and estimator parameters, a second experiment involving another patient was carried out. Figure 4.18 shows the result of the trial where it

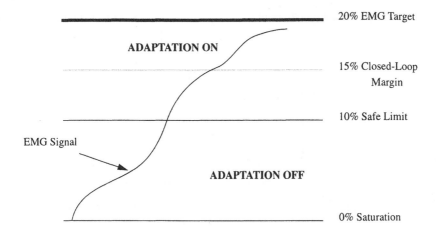

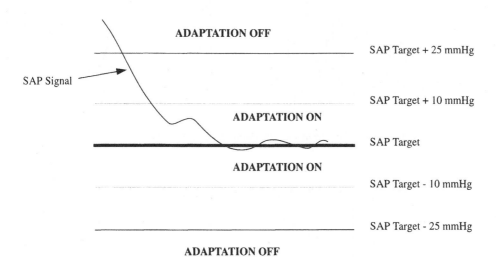

Figure 4.19   Diagram representing the EMG limits used for jacketing.

can be seen that the EMG signal was much closer to the 20% target than in the previous trial, except that at time 44 min the Relaxograph device started giving wrong readings due to heavy electrical interference, and as a result the closed-loop control was interrupted. Notice that in this case the SAP signal was less settled than in the previous case although the anaesthetist was satisfied with the overall performance.

Patient 3

For this experiment GPC had the following parameters:

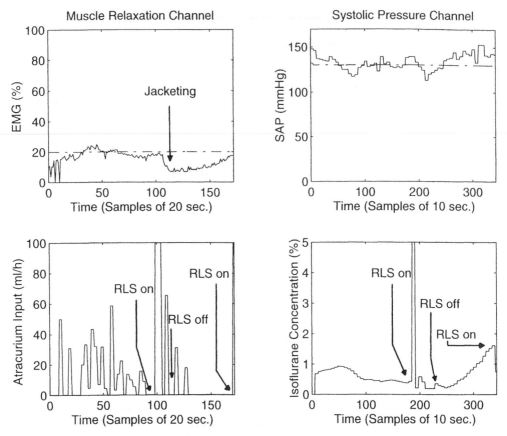

Figure 4.20   Performance of multivariable GPC during surgery for patient 3.

$$N_1 = 1; \quad N_2 = 10; \quad NU(\text{ch }1) = 2; \quad NU(\text{ch }2) = 1$$

$$\lambda = 0; \quad P = \begin{bmatrix} \dfrac{(1 - 0.7z^{-1})}{0.3} & 0 \\ 0 & \dfrac{(1 - 0.9z^{-1})}{0.1} \end{bmatrix}$$

$T(z^{-1}) = 1(1 - 0.85z^{-1})^2 I$ for control

$T(z^{-1}) = (1 - 0.80z^{-1})^2 I$ for estimation

This time, the idea behind the choice of the above tuning 'knobs' was to make the muscle relaxation channel relatively fast by increasing the number of degrees of freedom (with the obvious risk of a more activated control signal) and choosing a $P(z^{-1})$ such that the muscle relaxation channel is fast, but the blood pressure, which is the interactor channel, is slow. A form of 'jacketing' was devised according to the diagram of Figure 4.19, where the limits shown were considered to represent the safe regions of adaptive controller operation. As shown in Figure 4.20 the outputs in both channels tracked the set-points reasonably well until the 30th minute where the adaptation was switched on. At that time the blood pressure rose drastically due to surgical stimuli and the input responded with a high isoflurane input which in turn produced the interaction in the muscle relaxation channel which caused the switching off of the adaptation according to the jacketing policy of Figure 4.19. However, in response to a special questionnaire produced for each trial, the anaesthetist considered the trial performance to be good.

4.6 Conclusions

A multivariable model combining muscle relaxation and anaesthesia has been identified. The drugs atracurium and isoflurane were considered in the study. The system dynamics are of moderate complexity. This model complexity consists of a severe nonlinearity as well as large patient-to-patient variability in model parameters. It is because of the inability of fixed controllers to cope with controlling such systems (Linkens *et al.* 1982; Slate, 1980) that the use of adaptive control techniques was considered. The GPC algorithm which has been evaluated in the muscle relaxation SISO case both in simulations and clinical trials represented a very attractive candidate for the above task. The GPC extension to include the multivariable case was straightforward and the results show good performance in the examples of Figures 4.8–4.15. Control of relaxation was obviously harder than unconsciousness via blood pressure measurements. This was mainly due to the nonlinear pharmacodynamics. Results also demonstrated that in order to obtain smoother control actions, the basic algorithm needed to be extended to include the model-following polynomial $P(z^{-1})$, the observer polynomial $T(z^{-1})$, or both (Figures 4.12–4.15), especially if disturbances occur or the control horizon NU is taken greater than 1. Because the use of $P(z^{-1})$ affects both the disturbance rejection properties of the system as well as its overall closed-loop characteristics, it was possible to reach a trade-off relating stability and rise time between the two channels. As will be shown in subsequent chapters (Chapters 5 and 9), if the algorithm is modified to include input and output constraints as well as set-point pre-specification, even better results are possible.

The second part of the experiments considered devising a control system which could be transferred into theatre. The multivariable control system proved a very challenging process, since we had to make the computer communicate with four devices at each sampling time by making sure that it (the computer) reads two signals and delivers two signals successfully. In this difficult study we succeeded in conducting three trials where we were able to control muscle relaxation as well as systolic arterial pressure by on-line infusions of atracurium and isoflurane. These preliminary results were very encouraging from which various lessons can be learned:

1. As far as the muscle relaxation channel is concerned, we cannot afford to have an over-active channel by choosing a larger control horizon NU and a fast pole for the model-following polynomial.

2. A smoother approach to the set-point should be encouraged.

3. Some form of 'jacketing' is necessary to switch from the adaptive mode to the fixed mode, especially near the nonlinear zone (in our case when the EMG approaches 10%).

As far as blood pressure is concerned, it is widely agreed that the SAP variable is not easy to control due to various conditions independent of the feedback loop such as blood loss, patient's state of mind etc., but suffice to say that GPC managed to maintain the SAP signal within reasonable bounds acceptable to anaesthetists; it is worth noting here that when controlling blood pressure as an inferential variable to monitor unconsciousness it is not always necessary to obtain tight control, but a tolerance range is sufficient.

In the trial with Patient 2 we experienced the phenomenon of unreliable EMG measurements. This is a common phenomenon in operating theatres where electrical interference from surgical diathermy is quite frequent. To alleviate such problems it is necessary to superimpose an intelligent structure by adding a supervisory layer that monitors the variables involved (see Chapter 10). By doing this, the controller can fulfil successfully three tasks; namely control, adaptation and supervision.

Finally, the overall control system proved to be easy to manage by the anaesthetist, although further improvements in the hardware need to be introduced if the objective of the whole exercise is to relieve tedium for the anaesthetist. It is hoped to conduct further clinical trials in the future to assess the performance of the multivariable GPC over a wider range of patients, together with refinement of the protocols necessary to establish and maintain multivariable control for the majority of operating conditions.

CHAPTER FIVE

Constrained Multivariable Generalised Predictive Control for Anaesthesia: the Quadratic Programming Approach (QP)

5.1 Introduction

It is common knowledge that control constraints on system hardware are endemic, e.g. motors, valves etc. are all subject to limitations which the control algorithm must consider. A simple way of dealing with such limitations is to ignore them when solving the control objective and then clip the control sequence once it is calculated and memorise the clipped value for the next iteration. This methodology seems to work in practice, but the solution drifts further from the concept of *optimal solution*. Another way of solving this limiting problem is to include directly all the constraints within the control objective. Prett and Gillette (1980) proposed a method for including process constraints in the controller's cost function which they later applied to the optimal control of a Catalytic Cracking Unit. Garcia and Morshedi (1986) showed that input and output constraints could be formulated as linear inequality constraints. Tsang and Clarke (1988) considered such an approach within the SISO GPC structure and solved the problem by means of Lagrange multipliers and demonstrated that if input constraints were not explicitly included in the cost function minimisation problem, instability would occur for some system types and controller degrees of freedom. Recent work by Scokaert and Clarke (1994) focused on formulating stabilising properties relating to an earlier algorithm proposed by Clarke and Scattolini (1991), known as constrained receding horizon predictive control (CRHPC). This study, mainly concentrating on a SISO version, is particularly interesting as it tried to tackle the problem of incompatibility of constraints which is increasingly becoming a major area of interest in predictive control. Another study, due to Wilkinson *et al.* (1994), dealt with GPC and the linear quadratic programming (QP) approach as advocated by Lawson and Hanson (1974). The algorithm, which was applied to a distillation column model, shows great promise but the study did not include explicitly the merits of using either input constraints, output constraints or both.

In this chapter the QP approach is applied to the nonlinear anaesthesia multi-variable system comprising simultaneous control of muscle relaxation (paralysis) and anaesthesia (unconsciousness). The study concentrates first on the use of the unconstrained multivariable GPC followed by constrained multivariable GPC with input constraints (rate and magnitude), then constrained multivariable GPC with input and output constraints. All simulation experiments were conducted under deterministic and stochastic conditions. The study is divided into four sections. Section 5.2 is devoted to a brief description of the relationship between the GPC strategy and the least-squares problem. Section 5.3 is a series of simulation results obtained with the constrained GPC algorithm using the multivariable nonlinear anaesthesia model. Also, a comparative study between the algorithm that simply clips the control and the constrained algorithm is undertaken and the results obtained are analysed and discussed. Finally, in Section 5.4 conclusions are drawn with respect to the new algorithm, its power and limitations.

5.2 Theory of the constrained multivariable generalised predictive control

Several applications in applied mathematics, control theory and other fields require the standard 'least-squares' problem to be reformulated by the introduction of certain inequality constraints. These constraints constitute additional valuable information about the problem, without which the designed system would certainly not perform at its best. For instance, Garcia (1984) considered quadratic programming (QP) with the popular DMC algorithm and applied it to a batch reactor process and found it to perform extremely well. This ability to consider least-squares problems with linear inequality constraints allows us, in particular, to impose such constraints on the solution as non-negativity, or that each variable is to have independent upper and lower bounds, or that the sum of all the variables cannot exceed a specified value or that a fitted curve is to be monotone or convex.

Let A be an $m_2 \times n$ matrix, b an m_2 vector, C an $m \times n$ matrix, h an m vector.

The least-squares problem with linear inequality constraints can be stated as follows (Lawson and Hanson, 1974):

1. **LSI (least-squares inequality) problem**

    Minimise $\| Ax - b \|$ subject to $Cx > h$ (5.1)

    where x is the n solution vector, C the static/dynamic constraints information matrix and h a vector containing the lower and upper limits of the constraints.

    The following important special cases of the LSI problem will be considered:

2. **NNLS (non-negative least-squares) problem**

    Minimise $\| Ax - b \|$ subject to $Cx > 0$ (5.2)

3. **LDP (least-distance programming) problem**

    Minimise $\| x \|$ subject to $Cx > h$ (5.3)

Details of how to convert the LSI problem to the LDP problem (which is the most elegant way of tackling this category of problems) are given in Lawson and Hanson (1974) but are also summarised in Appendix III. However, the following shows briefly how to relate the multivariable GPC strategy to the quadratic programming (QP) approach.

Let us rewrite the cost function associated with GPC as the following expression:

$$J = (\omega - G_d u(t) - \Psi)^T (\omega - G_d u(t) - \Psi) + \Lambda u(t)^T u(t) \tag{5.4}$$

if

$$A = \begin{bmatrix} G_d \\ \Lambda^{1/2} \end{bmatrix}, \quad b = \begin{bmatrix} \omega - \Psi \\ 0 \end{bmatrix}$$

and $x = u$ then, minimising J would in effect be equivalent to minimising $\|Ax - b\|^2$ subject to $Cx \geq h$.

A is of dimension:

$$\begin{cases} m_1 \times n_1 \\ m_1 = \sum_{i=1}^{m} (N_{2i} - N_{1i} + 1) + \sum_{i=1}^{m} NU_i \\ n_1 = \sum_{i=1}^{m} NU_i \end{cases}$$

b is of dimension m_1, h is of dimension n_1.

The dimension of C depends on the type of constraints involved. Three types of constraints can be considered:

1. Input rate constraints.
2. Input magnitude constraints.
3. Output magnitude constraints.

The input rate constraints are usually expressed in terms of present and future control increment moves, i.e.:

$$\Delta u_{i\,\min} \leq \Delta u_i(t + j - 1) \leq \Delta u_{i\,\max}$$

$$i = 1, \ldots, m \tag{5.5}$$

$$j = 1, \ldots, NU_i$$

or

$$\Delta u_i(t + j - 1) \geq \Delta u_{i\,\min}$$

$$-\Delta u_i(t + j - 1) \geq -\Delta u_{i\,\max}$$

$$i = 1, \ldots, m$$

$$j = 1, \ldots, NU_i$$

$\Delta u_{i\,\min}$ and $\Delta \mu_{i\,\max}$ are the minimum and maximum allowed control increments respectively. In this particular case, the number of conditions generated in the constraint matrix C_0 is:

$$\left(\sum_{i=1}^{m} NU_i \right) \times 2$$

In turn, the input magnitude constraints are expressed in terms of the absolute control inputs, i.e.:

$$u_{i\,min} \leq u_i(t + j - 1) \leq u_{i\,max}$$

$$i = 1, \dots, m \tag{5.6}$$

$$j = 1, \dots, NU_i$$

In terms of Δu_i, equation (5.6) becomes:

$$u_{i\,min} \leq u_i(t) \leq u_{i\,max}$$

$$u_{i\,min} \leq u_i(t + 1) \leq u_{i\,max}$$

$$\vdots$$

$$u_{i\,min} \leq u_i(t + NU_i - 1) \leq u_{i\,max}$$

$$i = 1, \dots, m$$

or

$$u_{i\,min} - u(t - 1) \leq \Delta u_i(t) \leq u_{i\,max} - u(t - 1)$$

$$u_{i\,min} - u(t - 1) \leq \Delta u_i(t + 1) + \Delta u(t) \leq u_{i\,max} - u(t - 1)$$

$$\vdots$$

$$u_{i\,min} - u(t - 1) \leq \Delta u_i(t + NU_i - 1) + \Delta u_i(t + NU_i - 2) + \dots + \Delta u_i(t)$$

$$\leq u_{i\,max} - u(t - 1) \quad i = 1, \dots, m$$

which can also be written as the following:

$$\Delta u_i(t) \geq u_{i\,min} - u(t - 1)$$

$$-\Delta u_i(t) \geq -u_{i\,max} + u(t - 1)$$

$$\Delta u_i(t + 1) + \Delta u(t) \geq u_{i\,min} - u(t - 1)$$

$$-\Delta u_i(t + 1) - \Delta u(t) \geq -u_{i\,max} + u(t - 1)$$

$$\vdots$$

$$\Delta u_i(t + NU_i - 1) + \Delta u_i(t + NU_i - 2) + \dots + \Delta u_i(t) \geq u_{i\,min} - u(t - 1)$$

$$-\Delta u_i(t + NU_i - 1) - \Delta u_i(t + NU_i - 2) - \dots - \Delta u_i(t) \geq -u_{i\,max} + u(t - 1)$$

$$i = 1, \dots, m$$

$u_{i\,min}$ and $u_{i\,max}$ are the minimum and maximum allowed absolute control moves respectively. Also in this case, the number of conditions generated in the constraint matrix C_1 is:

$$\left(\sum_{i=1}^{m} NU_i \right) \times 2$$

Finally, output constraints can be included by using the future output predictions formulated in terms of past, present and future inputs as well as past and present outputs, i.e.:

$$\Phi_{i\,\min} \leq \Phi_i(t + j) \leq \Phi_{i\,\max}$$

$$j = 1, 2, \ldots, N_{2i} \tag{5.7}$$

$$i = 1, 2, \ldots, m$$

Φ_i min and Φ_i max are the minimum and maximum allowed outputs respectively. In this case, the number of conditions generated in the constraint matrix C_2 is:

$$\sum_{i=1}^{m} (N_{2i} - N_{1i} + 1) \times 2$$

Taking into account equation (4.25), equation (5.7) can written as:

$$\Phi_{\min} \leq (G_d U(t) + \Psi(t + j)) \leq \Phi_{\max}$$

$$j = N_{1i}, \ldots, N_{2i}$$

or

$$\Phi_{\min} - \Psi(t + j) \leq G_d U(t) \leq \Phi_{\max} - \Psi(t + j)$$

where $U(t)$ is the vector of control increments, which can also be written as the following:

$$G_d U(t) \geq \Phi_{\min} - \Psi(t + j)$$

$$-G_d U(t) \geq -\Phi_{\max} + \Psi(t + j)$$

If all three constraints are considered, then we would write the conditions as follows:

$$\Delta u_{i\,\min} \leq \Delta u_{i(t + j - 1)} \leq \Delta u_{i\,\max}$$

$$u_{i\,\min} \leq u_{i(t + j - 1)} \leq u_{i\,\max} \tag{5.8}$$

$$\Phi_{i\,\min} \leq \Phi_{i(t + j)} \leq \Phi_{i\,\max}$$

where $\Delta u_{i\,\min}$, $\Delta u_{i\,\max}$, $u_{i\,\min}$, $u_{i\,\max}$, $\Phi_{i\,\min}$ and $\Phi_{i\,\max}$ are the minimum and maximum allowed control increments, absolute control moves, and outputs respectively. It is worth noting that the third inequality in equation (5.8) can also be rewritten as the following:

$$\Phi_{\min} \leq (G_d u(t) + \Psi(t + j)) \leq \Phi_{\max}$$

$$j = N_{1i}, \ldots, N_{2i} \tag{5.9}$$

$$i = 1, \ldots, m$$

The overall dynamic constraint information matrix C will be equal to:

$$C = \begin{bmatrix} C_0 \\ C_1 \\ C_2 \end{bmatrix}$$

of dimension

$$\left(\left(\sum_{i=1}^{m} NU_i \right) \times 4 \right) + \left(\sum_{i=1}^{m} (N_{2i} - N_{1i} + 1) \right) \times 2$$

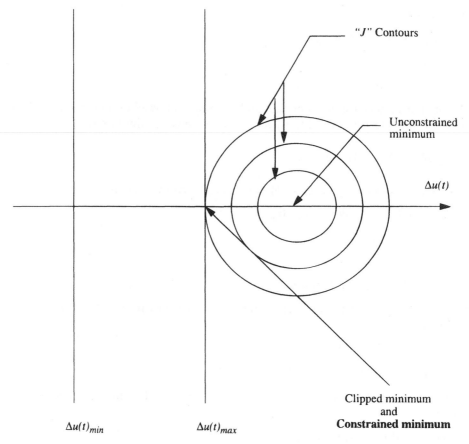

Figure 5.1   Position of the clipped and constrained minima for $NU = 1$.

The computational effort required to solve such an LSI problem increases with the number of constraint conditions included within the algorithm, especially when output magnitude constraints, whose number is linked to the output horizons N_{2i}, are included with those of input rate and input magnitude. It is therefore advisable to use double precision arithmetic calculations, and failure to do so would probably result in the algorithm failing to produce a solution to the optimisation problem.

5.2.1   The concept of feasibility

The issue of feasibility in optimisation is of utmost importance for it represents a bottleneck in deciding the failure or success of finding a solution to **hard** constraints in any optimising problem. This issue arises because of the possibility that when formulating inequality constraints on top of the cost function to be optimised, mutual **incompatibility** between the various constraint conditions arises preventing the optimiser from providing a projected control move; in other words the defined allowed region for the vector of postulated controls becomes empty (Scokaert, 1994;

Wilkinson *et al.*, 1994). Infeasibility in general can be viewed as follows. As shown in Figure 5.1 the '"*J*" = constant' contours are described by a set of circles whose common centre represents the unconstrained minimum control increment $\Delta u(t)*$ and where the clipped minimum as well as the constrained one are the same, while Figure 5.2 shows that for $NU = 2$ the '"*J*" = constant' contours are represented by a set of ellipses showing combinations of inputs giving the same value for the cost function. The two minima are different in this case. Constrained optimisation theory states that the constrained minimum of a function is given by the point at which the minimum diameter '*J*' contour just touches the constraint boundary. The closest ellipses can touch the constraint boundary from various positions (Tsang and Clarke, 1988). Feasibility problems can be divided into two types:

- *Type I infeasibilities.* These are caused mainly by equality and inequality constraints.
- *Type II infeasibilities.* These are caused by the fact that the optimiser cannot satisfy all inequality constraints and returns an empty region for the vector of

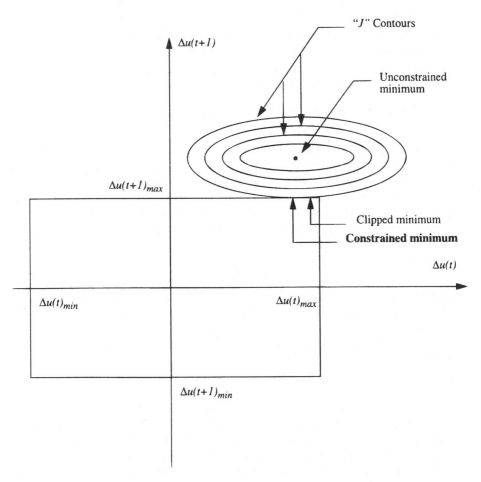

Figure 5.2 Position of the clipped and constrained minima for $NU = 2$.

postulated controls. This type of infeasibility, however, is rare when one type of constraint (input or output) is used at one time. It is, however, likely to occur when both types of constraints are used simultaneously especially in noise and disturbance contaminated environments, as occurs in the application considered in this chapter.

5.2.2 The handling of type II infeasibilities

Before proceeding further, one should first consider ways to prevent such infeasibility conditions occurring. Little is known about the causes of infeasibility as little research has hitherto been devoted to this subject despite calls from leading figures in optimisation, such as Morshedi *et al.* (1985) and Bortolotto and Jørgensen (1986), as noted by Scokaert (1994). However, there are a few points to take into consideration when dealing with inequality constraints:

1. When only input rate and input magnitude constraints are used, infeasibility is rare practically, either in the disturbed or undisturbed case. This is because noise and disturbances do not affect the manipulated variables.

2. The combination of input rate and input magnitude constraints with those of output magnitude leads to infeasibility of type II in the disturbed case.

3. A choice of a lower constraint horizon greater or equal to the constrained variable time delay reduces the likelihood of infeasibility.

In light of these considerations various alternatives exist for handling infeasibilities, of which two popular ones are:

1. **On-line switch to other forms of control**. Although this option is pragmatic in nature, it is the only alternative that one can use to avoid a complete shut-down of operation with the risk of jeopardising the normal operation of a system. In the case of optimisation, when failure to find a control solution due to incompatibility of inequality constraints occurs, one can switch to a more conservative control algorithm (fixed-term controller, unconstrained controller etc.), or alternatively pay the penalty of losing system accuracy by switching to manual control.

2. **Hierarchical constraints removal**. In contrast to **capitulation**, i.e. switch off the adaptive controller which uses constraints, one could try and remove some of the constraints that might be the cause of the clash between the input and output constraints. If a non-zero minimum time delay is considered in the control calculations, then the first constraint to remove is the one that corresponds to the submatrix $\bar{g}_{kj}$ in the dynamic step response matrix G_d whose four elements are zero (Mohtadi, 1986). Next, if the incompatibility still persists, then the constraints starting from the bottom of the predictions should be removed, since these are the ones the controller has least confidence in, especially in the presence of noise and disturbances (an analogy with weather forecasting can be made in this case). This process can be repeated until all the constraints are satisfied. **Capitulation** occurs when all output constraints are removed and only input constraints are left to **represent** the cost function. Figure 5.3 is a flow chart outlining the various steps involved in such a constraints removal mechanism.

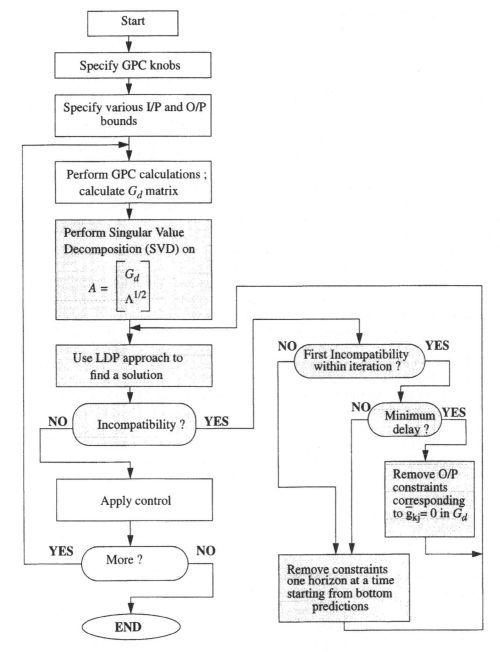

Figure 5.3 Flow chart representing the various steps involved in the hierarchical removal of output constraints.

Constraint relaxation is another way of dealing with incompatibility whereby less important constraints are gradually relaxed rather than removed. Although this method was successfully implemented with the DMC approach, it will not be dealt with in this study.

5.3   Simulation results

The simulation study considered the continuous nonlinear multivariable anaesthetic model for simultaneous control of unconsciousness and muscle relaxation using multiple drug administration similar to the one used in Chapter 4 and described by equation (4.14). Conditions for simulation are similar to the ones adopted in Chapter 4. For parameter estimation, a UD factorisation method was used on incremental data with the initial covariance matrix and forgetting factor given by: $Cov = 10^2. I$ and $\rho = 0.975$ respectively. In the multivariable GPC case, a multivariable model of 5 diagonal $A(z^{-1})$ matrices together with 5 upper triangular $B(z^{-1})$ matrices was estimated (Linkens and Mahfouf, 1994). Initial conditions were 0% relaxation and 100 mmHg arterial pressure. The set-point command signal was 0.80 for relaxation, and 80 mmHg followed by 70 mmHg periodically for the blood pressure. A bolus u_1 of atracurium of 67 mg at 1 mg ml^{-1} concentration was initially applied for one sample and input u_2 was kept at 0. While the bolus effect persisted, the loop remained open until the output in the muscle relaxation channel reached the safety level of 0.85 at which point the loop was closed, this protocol being similar to the one used by anaesthetists in theatre and which also enables the surgeon to initiate surgery as quickly as possible. The GPC algorithm was allowed to run with some initial parameter estimates, which were obtained at the end of a trial run using the unconstrained multivariable GPC algorithm, until sample time 41 min at which time the parameter estimation routine was made to be operational. Two disturbances were simulated at different times; the first one in the form of an output disturbance of 20 mmHg at time 180 min lasting for 5 minutes in the blood pressure channel and which mimics various surgical stimuli, while the second was in the form of an open-loop gain change from 1 to 2.5 at time 350 min in the muscle relaxation channel and lasting for 100 minutes and which corresponds to a variation in the patient's sensitivity to the drug caused by blood loss. The GPC tuning knobs were set to $N_1 = 1$, $N_2 = 7$, $NU_1 = 2$, $NU_2 = 1$, $\Lambda = 0$, $P(z^{-1}) = I$. For the polynomial matrix $T(z^{-1})$, we selected the diagonal elements to be second order of the form:

$$T(z^{-1}) = \begin{bmatrix} (1 - 0.7z^{-1})^2 & 0 \\ 0 & (1 - 0.7z^{-1})^2 \end{bmatrix}$$

for control and for estimation. The use of second order filters was found to add more robustness when rejecting disturbances and it also compensates for unmodelled dynamics more effectively (Mohtadi, 1989).

The study was divided into three parts: the first part concerned the use of the multivariable GPC algorithm with clipped input signals, while the second part included the input rate and input magnitude constraints with the following limiting values:

$$\Delta u_{1\,min} = -0.10, \ \Delta u_{1\,max} = 0.10, \ \Delta u_{2\,min} = -0.10, \ \Delta u_{2\,max} = 0.10$$

and

$$u_{1\,min} = 0, \ u_{1\,max} = 1, \ u_{2\,min} = 0, \ u_{2\,max} = 5$$

Finally, the third series of the experiments considered a combination of input rate and input magnitude constraints together with output magnitude constraints having the following output limits (for MAP the values represent absolute values rather than changes):

$$\Phi_{1\,min} = 0.78, \; \Phi_{1\,max} = 0.82, \; \Phi_{2\,min} = 67 \text{ mmHg}, \; \Phi_{2\,max} = 100 \text{ mmHg}$$

5.3.1 Simulations in a noise-free environment

The multivariable GPC algorithm with clipped control

In this series of experiments the control signals $u_1(t)$ and $u_2(t)$, obtained by minimising the cost function (5.4), were simply clipped between the minimum and maximum already specified, i.e. $0 \leq u_1(t) \leq 1$ and $0 \leq u_2(t) \leq 5$. Figure 5.4 shows that the algorithm did not demonstrate any unstable modes but there were large control excursions especially during the disturbance phases. It should be noted that a saturating signal in the first channel together with the large drop in the blood pressure at time 180 min would be considered to be a serious risk to patients in operating theatres. Notice that after the output disturbance in the blood pressure channel, the response seems to be slow at tracking the set-point change, this being

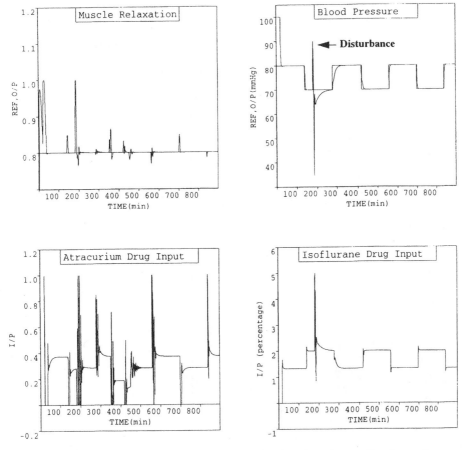

Figure 5.4 Multivariable GPC of the anaesthesia model in the 'clipped control' and noise-free case: $NU_1 = 2$, $NU_2 = 1$ and with $T(z^{-1})$.

due to the fact that the parameter estimates were detuned. However, once enough excitation has been provided, the parameter estimates improved and set-point tracking was better.

Input rate and input magnitude constraints

Figure 5.5 shows the result of a run where it can be seen that the above constraints with respect to the control moves were all satisfied producing a tighter control especially in the paralysis channel which is the channel affected by interactions. The slight kick in the blood pressure channel at time 350 min is due to the abrupt large change in the open-loop gain introduced in the paralysis channel. Although the system is triangular, implying that one channel only is affected by interactions, in closed-loop control interactions can occur in both channels (Mohtadi *et al.*, 1992).

Input rate, input magnitude and output constraints

For this series of experiments, output constraints were combined with those of input rate and input magnitude constraints. A typical run produced the performance shown in Figure 5.6a where it can be seen that, as expected, the algorithm produced

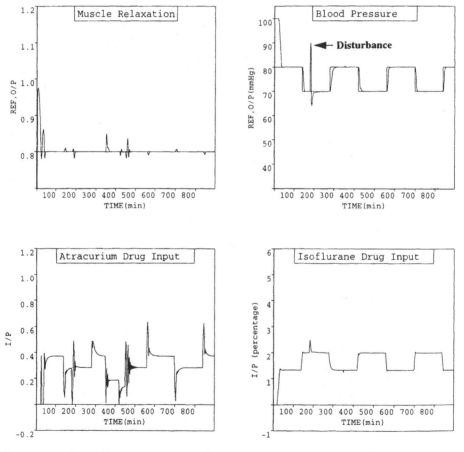

Figure 5.5 Multivariable constrained GPC of the anaesthesia model with input rate and input magnitude constraints in the noise-free case: $NU_1 = 2$, $NU_2 = 1$.

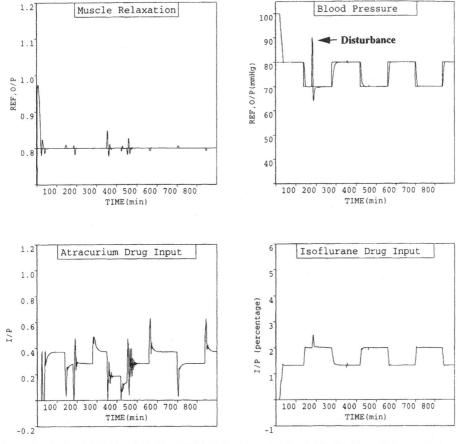

Figure 5.6a Multivariable constrained GPC of the anaesthesia model with input and output constraints in the noise-free case: $NU_1 = 2$, $NU_2 = 1$.

an equally tight control in the muscle relaxation channel as in the previous run. Also, the outputs were kept within the specified limiting values. This is also apparent from Figure 5.6b where the number of output constraints ignored is plotted against time. However, it is only when the loop was closed for the first time and at the occurrence time of the disturbances that the algorithm reverted back to the input rate and input magnitude constraints after a series of hierarchical output constraints removal. It is also interesting to note that at times nearing 30 minutes and 200 minutes only the constraint conditions corresponding to $\bar{g}_{1k} = 0$ (the first $4k$ elements in the dynamic step response matrix, k being the time delay) were removed since the number of output constraints ignored was 4, confirming the point made earlier in the section relating to the hierarchical constraints removal (see Section 5.2.2).

5.3.2   Simulation in a noise-contaminated environment

Throughout this next series of simulations, noise sequences of 1% and 5 mmHg peak for the muscle relaxation and blood pressure channels respectively were considered.

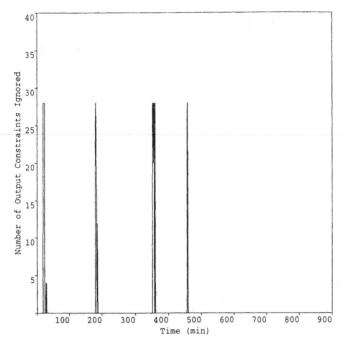

Figure 5.6b   Number of output constraints removed for the run corresponding to Figure 5.6a.

The multivariable GPC algorithm with clipped control

Figure 5.7 shows the output performances of the multivariable GPC with clipped control. As with Figure 5.4, large control excursions can be seen during the disturbance phases in both channels together with a saturating paralysis signal and a large drop in the blood pressure signal.

Input rate and input magnitude constraints

As in the similar section, Section 5.3.1, a series of experiments using the input rate and input magnitude constraints was carried out. Figure 5.8 shows the output performance of the algorithm. All disturbances were successfully dealt with without violating the various input bounds.

Input rate, input magnitude and output constraints

In the final part of the experiments, input constraints were combined with those of output constraints in a noise-contaminated environment. The experiment produced the output performances of Figure 5.9a which, if compared to those of Figure 5.8, are visually similar. This can be explained by the fact that at the time of disturbances the algorithm, not being able to satisfy all constraints, removed all output constraints and reverted to the output constraints algorithm, as can be seen from the number of output constraints removed as shown in Figure 5.9b. Also, in the same

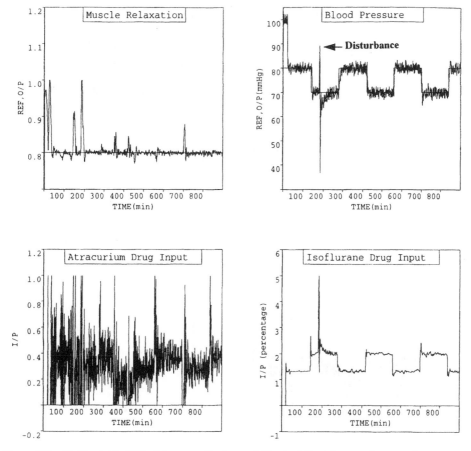

Figure 5.7 Multivariable GPC of the anaesthesia model in the 'clipped control' case and noise-contaminated environment: $NU_1 = 2$, $NU_2 = 1$.

figure it can be seen that at times 400, 450, and 560 the algorithm only removed the output constraints corresponding to $\bar{g}_{1k} = 0$. It is also worth mentioning that a close examination of the blood pressure channel leads one to conclude that it has been slowed down slightly (especially at the beginning of the run), and this can be explained by the fact that by adding the output constraints, the algorithm with its *hard* constraining policy tries to sacrifice some of its performance in the second channel to reduce the level of interactions in the first channel (hard constraints imply that the algorithm has to satisfy the conditions of any cost).

5.3.3 A comparative study of the different constraining regimes

In order to complement the visual indications of control performance from these experiments, an objective measure of performance over the simulation runs was made using ISE (integral of square errors) criterion. The study included experiments

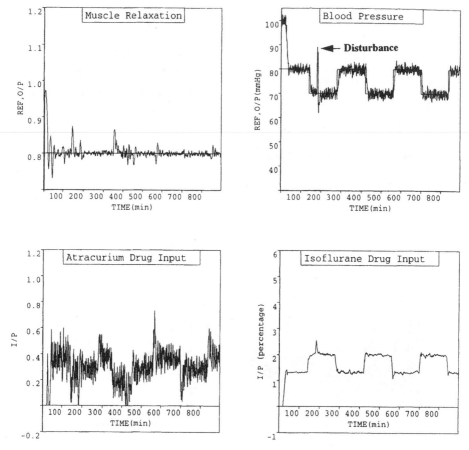

Figure 5.8 Multivariable constrained GPC of the anaesthesia model with input rate and input magnitude constraints with a noise-contaminated environment: $NU_1 = 2$, $NU_2 = 1$.

that are not possible to show because of lack of space, especially those that considered control horizons of $NU_1 = NU_2 = 1$ and we refer to them as *Not shown*. Table 5.1 gives the ISE values for the various channels in the deterministic case, whereas Table 5.2 gives these criteria in the stochastic case (the ISE values in the blood pressure channel have been scaled down by a factor of 1000).

In the deterministic case, as shown in Table 5.1 lower ISE values were obtained in the muscle relaxation channel with the constrained algorithm, the lowest of which was that obtained with the algorithm including both input and output constraints with control horizons of $NU_1 = 2$, $NU_2 = 1$ and corresponding to Figure 5.6a (ISE = 0.0248). In order to realise such performance, the algorithm had to sacrifice some of its performance in the blood pressure channel, which was model interaction free. In other words, the algorithm directed most of its hard constraining job to the channel that bears all the interactions, i.e. the muscle relaxation channel. The 'kicks' observed in that channel bear witness to this, despite the fact that the system is triangular. Moreover, when a disturbance sends the output above the set-point then

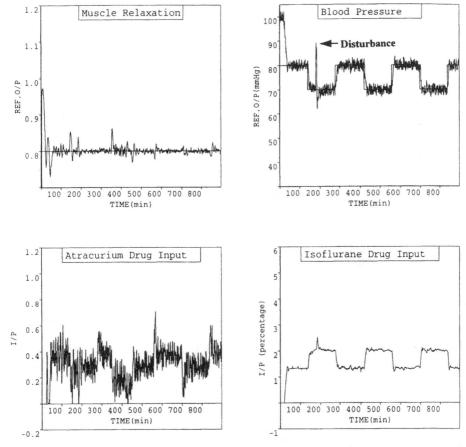

Figure 5.9a Multivariable constrained GPC of the anaesthesia model with input and output constraints with a noise-contaminated environment: $NU_1 = 2$, $NU_2 = 1$.

back the other way within a relatively short time, it is likely to produce smaller ISEs than when the same output is kept within reasonable bounds at the cost of a slower recovery from the disturbance.

Again, in the stochastic case (Table 5.2), the lowest ISE in the muscle relaxation channel was obtained with the algorithm using the input and output constraints with control horizons of $NU_1 = 2$ and $NU_2 = 1$ (Figure 5.9a). As far as the muscle relaxation channel was concerned, the inclusion of output constraints produced better criteria than the case without the output constraints. It is true that the output constraints were not all satisfied all the time and there were instances where they were hierarchically removed from the algorithm but the performance overall was better than when the output constraints were not considered. Following the experiments carried out above and many more which cannot be shown here, it has been noticed that disturbances in the form of set-point changes did not seem to cause infeasibility, but those in the form of abrupt output and gain changes caused the algorithm to consider only input constraints until the disturbance was totally rejected. This, in our opinion, is due to several factors:

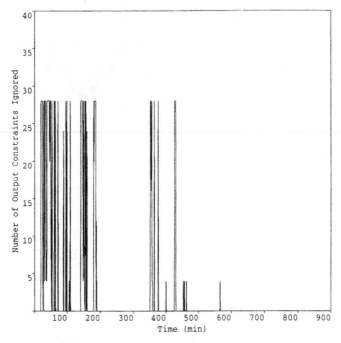

Figure 5.9b   Number of output constraints removed for the run corresponding to Figure 5.9a.

Table 5.1   ISE criteria for experiments in the deterministic case

Figure number	Type of algorithm	Muscle relaxation ISE	Blood pressure ISE
Not shown	Multivariable GPC with clipped control; $NU_1 = NU_2 = 1$	0.6867	0.6301
5.4	Multivariable GPC with clipped control; $NU_1 = 2; NU_2 = 1$	0.6462	0.6301
Not shown	Constrained multivariable GPC with input constraints; $NU_1 = NU_2 = 1$	0.0708	0.7952
5.5	Constrained multivariable GPC with input constraints; $NU_1 = 2; NU_2 = 1$	0.0495	0.7950
Not shown	Constrained multivariable GPC with input and output constraints; $NU_1 = NU_2 = 1$	0.0552	0.8058
5.6A	Constrained multivariable GPC with input and output constraints; $NU_1 = 2; NU_2 = 1$	0.0248	0.8187

Table 5.2   ISE criteria for experiments in the stochastic case

Figure number	Type of algorithm	Muscle relaxation ISE	Blood pressure ISE
Not shown	Multivariable GPC with clipped control; $NU_1 = NU_2 = 1$	0.8183	0.7808
5.7	Multivariable GPC with clipped control; $NU_1 = 2; NU_2 = 1$	0.7687	0.7808
Not shown	Constrained multivariable GPC with input constraints; $NU_1 = NU_2 = 1$	0.1917	0.9455
5.8	Constrained multivariable GPC with input constraints; $NU_1 = 2; NU_2 = 1$	0.1667	0.9455
Not shown	Constrained multivariable GPC with input and output constraints; $NU_1 = NU_2 = 1$	0.1455	0.9965
5.9A	Constrained multivariable GPC with input and output constraints; $NU_1 = 2; NU_2 = 1$	0.1370	0.9476

1. The output predictions become less credible at the time of the disturbance; the use of the observer polynomial $T(z^{-1})$ can help considerably providing that its roots are chosen appropriately (Mohtadi, 1989).

2. The addition of more constraints does not necessarily produce an optimal control move, especially in a noisy environment, and it means that the controller has to give up some performance in one channel (i.e. slow it down) to reduce interactions in the other.

5.4   Conclusions

Model-based predictive control (MBPC) and particularly the theme of GPC has in the last eight years shaped adaptive control research in such a way that it has convinced many sceptics in industry as well as in the life sciences that this form of control is safe and generally performs satisfactorily. It owes its popularity to its 'easy and elegant to implement' formulation and also to key control objectives which make it possible to include any constraints the system might be imposing. While many successful applications have been reported using the unconstrained algorithm (Lambert, 1987a; Mahfouf *et al.*, 1992), only a few have been reported using a version that includes the constraints in the cost function (Wilkinson *et al.*, 1994; Kwok *et al.*, 1991). A review of the various research work hitherto carried out in the domain of generalised predictive control and optimisation has suggested taking the GPC algorithm and superimposing the constraints on top of the cost function in order to solve the problem (Tsang and Clarke, 1988; Wilkinson *et al.*, 1994). In this study, we chose to conserve the GPC structure and include the quadratic programming (QP) approach developed by Lawson and Hanson (1974). The reason for this choice was the fact that the numerical and convergence properties of such an approach are good, and also it can in most cases guarantee optimality of the solution, despite the fact that it is computationally intensive. As outlined in the previous sections, various constraints can be accommodated easily, i.e. input rate, input magnitude, and output magnitude constraints. In the series of simulations carried out using the multivariable anaesthesia model, it has been shown that while the unconstrained algorithm did not display any unstable modes in the face of heavy disturbances, the control excursions were unacceptably large and it also showed poor set-point tracking properties. When constraints were included in the cost function, the performance was generally better in terms of disturbance rejection and set-point tracking despite the use of a relatively low output prediction N_2 which usually leads to fast feedback characteristics. In further experiments carried out but not shown here, it was possible to use an output prediction horizon N_2 as low as 5 with the constrained algorithm still giving a good performance but the unconstrained one produced ringing modes in the control signal when the output disturbances in the blood pressure channel occurred. In addition, the control activity was less extensive, a factor which is crucial in biomedicine ensuring that no unnecessary drug is administered to the patient. In general, it was found that the combination of input and output constraints gives more robustness to the whole structure although the likelihood of infeasibility increases. However, a solution is always guaranteed by the algorithm reverting to input constraints type only after hierarchical removal of the constraints thought to cause the infeasibility. Obviously, while the algorithm is carrying out this removal process, the processing time is bound to increase, but as far as the anaesthesia process which includes relatively slow dynamics, sampling times are in the order of 1 minute, giving adequate time for the algorithm to find a solution. In fact, the algorithm was implemented on SUN SPARC station and took a maximum of 3 seconds to complete one iteration.

The present study included simulation results where all types of constraints, i.e. input magnitude, input rate and output magnitude constraints, were used simultaneously. This allows better assessment of the robustness of the algorithm as far as the concept of feasibility is concerned, an issue which has not received due attention in the papers which dealt with the QP approach and which were mentioned previously. The results obtained in this study are very encouraging and give confidence in its clinical and other process feasibility.

CHAPTER SIX

Generalised Predictive Control with Feedforward (GPCF) for Multivariable Anaesthesia

6.1 Introduction

The development and application of GPC to SISO muscle relaxation has been validated in a series of clinical trials as seen in Chapter 2. In Chapter 4 SISO GPC has been extended to include simultaneous control of muscle relaxation and unconsciousness via blood pressure measurements in operating theatre via its multivariable version (MIMO GPC). Through these studies, considerable expertise has been gained in the selection of the design parameters which are inherent in GPC. As already seen in Chapter 4, the selection of design parameters is considerably more difficult in the MIMO case, and one possibility is to use a decoupling precompensator and then to apply individual SISO GPC controllers to each loop. This has further design burdens and does not necessarily give good disturbance rejection.

Another possibility is that generalised predictive control with feedforward (GPCF) can be developed for the MIMO case under certain model restrictions (Lee *et al.*, 1991). The anaesthetic model which is one-way interactive fulfils these restricted conditions. GPCF offers advantages and simplicity in design, improved transient and disturbance performance, together with highly reduced computational burden. These matters are investigated in this chapter via comparative simulation studies encompassing GPC in feedback and feedforward modes. Relative advantages of the two approaches are discussed.

6.2 Multivariable GPC with feedforward

Many processes have additive disturbances which are measurable. With interacting processes the disturbances in one loop may be controlled variables of other loops. These measurable disturbances added to the model structure in a feedforward manner can be considered as noise affecting the output. The more accurate is the model of the process, the better the predictive model becomes and hence, the variance of the measured output is reduced, and in this case, the controlled behaviour is improved (Clarke, 1985). As many feedforward terms as required can be included, and by using variables from other loops the interaction between loops can be reduced (Astrom and Wittenwark, 1989). In a multivariable context, a P-canonical structure as advocated by Kam *et al.* (1985) would be more appropriate since in this particular case loop interactions are treated as feedforward couplings. Changes in one transfer element influence only the corresponding output. The particular advantages offered by the use of this structure include the possibility of estimating the delays within the path (important in the GMV case) and also the fact that the number of inputs is not necessarily equal to the number of outputs in contrast to the V-canonical form. However, given the nature of the model for anaesthesia considered in this chapter which includes only one significant interaction path, the scheme which consists of using two single loop controllers and incorporating feedforward in one of the loops for the interaction is a sufficient technique.

The main idea of this controller is as follows: an *m*-input and *m*-output MIMO system can be represented by *m* SISO loops with interactions within the MIMO system considered as measurable disturbances to each of the SISO loops. In order to develop the multivariable GPC algorithm with feedforward, it is necessary to formulate first the algorithm relative to the SISO GPC algorithm (Clarke *et al.*, 1987a, 1987b) but including feedforward.

6.2.1   SISO GPC with feedforward

Similarly to Section 2.4, consider the following locally linearised discrete model in the backward shift operator z^{-1}:

$$A(z^{-1})y(t) = B(z^{-1})u(t-1) + D(z^{-1})v(t-1) + x(t) \tag{6.1}$$

where

$$A(z^{-1}) = 1 + a_1 z^{-1} + a_2 z^{-2} + \ldots + a_n z^{-n}$$

$$B(z^{-1}) = z^{-k}(b_1 + b_2 z^{-1} + b_3 z^{-2} + \ldots + b_m z^{-m+1})$$

$$D(z^{-1}) = z^{-kv}(d_1 + d_2 z^{-1} + d_3 z^{-2} + \ldots + d_d z^{-d+1})$$

and $y(t)$ is the measured variable; $u(t)$ the control input; k the assumed value of time delay; $v(t)$ the measured feedforward signal; k_v the assumed value of time delay in the feedforward term.

Similarly to Section 2.4, $x(t)$ represents the disturbance upon which the model is based and is considered to be of moving average form, i.e.:

$$x(t) = C(z^{-1}) \frac{\xi(t)}{\Delta} \tag{6.2}$$

where

$$C(z^{-1}) = c_0 + c_1 z^{-1} + c_2 z^{-2} + \ldots + c_p z^{-p}$$

$$\xi(t) = \text{an uncorrelated random sequence}$$

$$\Delta = 1 - z^{-1}$$

Thus, substituting equation (6.2) into equation (6.1) and appending the operator Δ gives:

$$A(z^{-1})\Delta y(t) = B(z^{-1})\Delta u(t-1) + D(z^{-1})\Delta v(t-1) + C(z^{-1})\xi(t) \tag{6.3}$$

The controller therefore computes the vector of controls using optimisation of a function having a similar form given by equation (2.12), i.e.:

$$\begin{cases} J = [(Q1 + Q2)] \\ Q1 = \sum_{j=N_1}^{N_2} [(P(z^{-1})\hat{y}(t+j) - \omega(t+j))^2] \\ Q2 = \sum_{j=1}^{NU} [\lambda(j)(\Delta u(t+j-1))^2] \end{cases} \tag{6.4}$$

However, because the feedforward term is now being included, the following variable definitions are considered:

$$P\hat{y}(t+j) = \bar{\bar{G}}_j \Delta u(t+j-1) + \Psi(t+j) \tag{6.5}$$

$$\Psi(t+j) = \bar{G}_j \Delta u^f(t-1) + \bar{F}_j y^f(t) + S_j \Delta v^f(t+j-1) \tag{6.6}$$

$$S_j = E_j D \quad \text{and} \quad \Delta v(t+j-1) = 0 \quad \text{for } j \geq 2 \tag{6.7}$$

Similarly to Section 2.4, the minimisation of the cost function described in equation (6.4) leads to the following projected control increment:

$$\Delta u(t) = \bar{g}^T(\omega - \Psi) \tag{6.8}$$

For the control (6.8) to be causal, the condition $k \leq k_v$ must be satisfied: this implies that the input $u(t)$ is likely to act faster (or at the same time) on the output $y(t)$ than the signal $v(t)$ (Lee *et al.*, 1991).

6.2.2 The GPCF algorithm

Now, the same technique can be modified to be applied to multivariable systems. Thus, consider the dual-input dual-output system of the form:

$$\begin{aligned} A_1(z^{-1})y_1(t) &= B_1(z^{-1})u_1(t-1) + D_1(z^{-1})u_2(t-1) + \frac{C_1(z^{-1})}{\Delta}\zeta_1(t) \\ A_2(z^{-1})y_2(t) &= B_2(z^{-1})u_2(t-1) + D_2(z^{-1})u_1(t-1) + \frac{C_2(z^{-1})}{\Delta}\zeta_2(t) \end{aligned} \tag{6.9}$$

where

$$A_i(z^{-1}) = 1 + a_{i0}z^{-1} + a_{i1}z^{-2} + \ldots + a_{inai}z^{-nai}$$

$$B_i(z^{-1}) = z^{-kii}(b_{i1} + b_{i2}z^{-1} + \ldots + b_{inbi}z^{-nbi+1})$$

$$D_i(z^{-1}) = z^{-kim}(d_{i1} + d_{i2}z^{-1} + \ldots + d_{indi}z^{-ndi+1})$$

$$C_i(z^{-1}) = c_{i0} + c_{i1}z^{-1} + c_{i2}z^{-2} \ldots + c_{inci}z^{-nci}$$

$$1 \leq i \leq 2, 1 \leq m \leq 2 \quad \text{and} \quad i \neq m$$

In the above, it is assumed that u_1 is the input which is most strongly correlated with y_1, and u_2 is the other input which is the most strongly correlated with y_2. In practice, this is equivalent to saying that u_1 is the signal that influences y_1 with the least time delay in channel 1. The same situation applies in channel 2.

Summarising leads to the following double inequality:

$$k_{11} \leq k_{12}$$
$$k_{22} \leq k_{21}$$

(6.10)

Using equation (6.8), the following control laws can be obtained for the two different channels:

$$\Delta u_i(t) = \bar{g}_i^T(\omega_i - \Psi_i) \quad \text{for } 1 \leq i \leq 2$$

(6.11)

where

$$\Psi_i = [\Psi_i(t + N_1), \dots, \Psi_i(t + N_2)] \quad \text{for } 1 \leq i \leq 2$$

In the above it is assumed that the GPC tuning knobs are identical for both channels, although these can be chosen to be different if necessary (Mahfouf, 1991).

Using equation (6.6) and taking $N_1 = 1$ without loss of generality, it follows that:

$$\Psi_i(t + 1) = \bar{G}_{i1}\Delta u_i^f(t - 1) + \bar{F}_{i1} y_i^f(t) + S_{i1}\Delta u_m^f(t)$$
$$\vdots$$
$$\Psi_i(t + N_2) = \bar{G}_{iN_2} \Delta u_i^f(t - 1) + \bar{F}_{iN_2} y_i^f(t) + S_{iN_2} \Delta u_m^f(t + N_2 - 1)$$

(6.12)

$$1 \leq i, m \leq 2 \quad \text{and} \quad i \neq m$$

with $\Delta u_m(t + j - 1) = 0 \ (j \geq 2)$ and $S_{ij} = E_j D_i \ (1 \leq j \leq N_2)$.

Making the increments at time t relating to the feedforward term appear in the above expressions leads to:

$$\Psi_i(t + 1) = \bar{G}_{i1}\Delta u_i^f(t - 1) + \bar{F}_{i1} y_i^f(t) + (S_{i1} - s_{i1})\Delta u_m^f(t) + s_{i1}\Delta u_m^f(t)$$
$$\vdots$$
$$\Psi_i(t + N_2) = \bar{G}_{iN_2} \Delta u_i^f(t - 1) + \bar{F}_{iN_2} y_i^f(t) + (S_{iN_2} - s_{iN_2} z^{-N_2+1})\Delta u_m^f(t + N_2 - 1) + s_{iN_2}\Delta u_m^f(t)$$

(6.13)

$$1 \leq i, m \leq 2 \quad \text{and} \quad i \neq m$$

with $\Delta u_m(t + j - 1) = 0$ for $j \geq 2$, or:

$$\Psi_i(t + j) = \bar{\Psi}_i(t + j) + s_{ij} \Delta u_m^f(t)$$
$$1 \leq j \leq N_2, 1 \leq i, m \leq 2 \quad \text{and} \quad i \neq m$$

(6.14)

Taking into account equations (6.11) and (6.14) yields:

$$\Delta u_1(t) + \bar{g}_1^T \bar{S}_1 \Delta u_2^f(t) = \bar{g}_1^T(\omega_1 - \Psi_1)$$
$$\Delta u_2(t) + \bar{g}_2^T \bar{S}_2 \Delta u_1^f(t) = \bar{g}_2^T(\omega_2 - \Psi_2)$$

(6.15)

with

$$\Delta u_2(t + j - 1) = 0 \quad \text{for } j \geq 2$$
$$\Delta u_1(t + j - 1) = 0 \quad \text{for } j \geq 2$$

and where $\bar{S}_1$ and $\bar{S}_2$ are vectors of the following form:

$$\bar{S}_i^T = [s_{i1}, s_{i2}, \ldots, s_{iN_2}] \quad \text{for } 1 \leq i \leq 2$$

In the case of the time delays (k_{12} and k_{21}) in the feedforward elements being different from zero, the leading k_{12} and k_{21} coefficients of $\bar{S}_1$ and $\bar{S}_2$ respectively are taken to be zero.

Thus, it can be seen that the values of the control signals relating to the two channels can then be obtained by solving the system equations (6.15) simultaneously. For reference purposes, this multivariable self-tuning controller will be referred to throughout as the MIMO generalised predictive controller incorporating feedforward (**GPCF**). It is worth noting, however, that in the case of the multivariable anaesthetic model, the solution of the previous system is considerably reduced since the second interaction which would affect the blood pressure path is absent, and when implemented, the scheme would consist of calculating the second control sequence Δu_2 first from the first equation in (6.15), then substituting its present and past (possibly filtered) values in the second equation to obtain the value of Δu_1 as the following system equations show:

$$\Delta u_1(t) + \bar{g}_1^T \bar{S}_1 \Delta u_2^f(t) = \bar{g}_1^T(\omega_1 - \bar{\Psi}_1)$$
$$\Delta u_2(t) = \bar{g}_2^T(\omega_2 - \bar{\Psi}_2)$$

(6.16)

where

$$\bar{\Psi}_2(t+1) = \bar{G}_{21}\Delta u_2^f(t-1) + \bar{F}_{21}\, y_2^f(t)$$

$$\vdots$$

$$\bar{\Psi}_2(t+N_2) = \bar{G}_{2N_2}\Delta u_2^f(t-1) + \bar{F}_{2N_2}\, y_2^f(t)$$

and

$$\Delta u_2(t+j-1) = 0 \quad \text{for } j \geq 2$$

At this stage it is worth noting that in order to fulfil the condition $\Delta u_i(t+j-1) = 0$ for $j \geq 2$, i being the ith channel, it is necessary to eliminate all elements in equation (6.16) which include those future control increments.

6.3 Simulation results

The simulation studies have been undertaken in two parts, the first part being concerned with validating the GPCF algorithm using the nonlinear multivariable anaesthetic model described in Chapter 4, the second consisted of conducting a comparative study with the multivariable GPC algorithm using a P-canonical structure of the estimated model (Linkens *et al.*, 1991). The nonlinear anaesthetic multivariable model was simulated using a fourth-order Runge–Kutta method with fixed step length for the integration. The study used a step length of 0.1 and a sampling interval of 1 minute. Initial conditions were 0% relaxation and 140 mmHg arterial pressure. The set-point command signal was 80% then 70% every 100 samples for relaxation, and 110 mmHg then 120 mmHg every 140 samples for blood pressure unless otherwise specified.

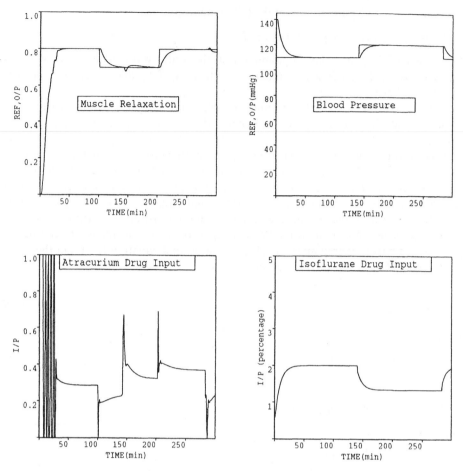

Figure 6.1   Extended GPCF algorithm with $P(z^{-1})$; $N_1 = 1$; $N_2 = 10$; $NU = 2$; $P_1 = P_2 = 10(1 - 0.9z^{-1})$.

During the first 25 samples initial control was provided by the GPC algorithm but with fixed parameter estimates obtained from the nominal linear model. The input signal was limited between 0 and 1.0 for the atracurium drug input, and between 0% and 5% for the isoflurane input. For parameter estimation, a UD-factorisation method (Bierman, 1977) was used on incremental data, with a forgetting factor and an initial covariance matrix given by:

$$\rho = 0.995 \quad \text{and} \quad Cov = 10^2.I$$

I being the identity matrix.

6.3.1   Experiments with the GPCF algorithm

A third-order model with a time delay of 1 minute and with two coefficients for the feedforward was considered for the first channel (muscle relaxation), whereas for the

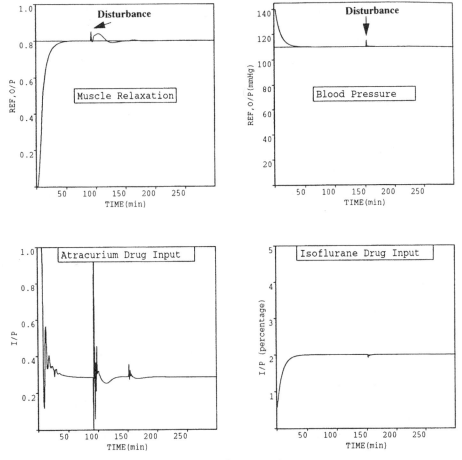

Figure 6.2 Extended GPCF algorithm with $P(z^{-1})$ and $T(z^{-1})$; $N_1 = 1$; $N_2 = 10$; $NU = 2$; $P_1 = P_2 = 10(1 - 0.9z^{-1})$ and $T_1 = T_2 = 1 - 0.9z^{-1}$.

second channel (blood pressure), a first model also with a 1 minute time delay was considered. The experiments were conducted in three phases, with sample results as follows.

Phase 1

Figure 6.1 shows a result from phase 1 where the controller parameter settings were identical for both channels:

$$N_1 = 1, \quad N_2 = 10, \quad NU = 2, \quad T(z^{-1}) = 1 \quad \text{and} \quad P(z^{-1}) = \frac{1 - 0.9z^{-1}}{0.1}$$

The idea behind this particular choice was to use a high value for the control horizon NU and modify the set-point responses by including the important model-following polynomial $P(z^{-1})$, parameters of which were selected based on the

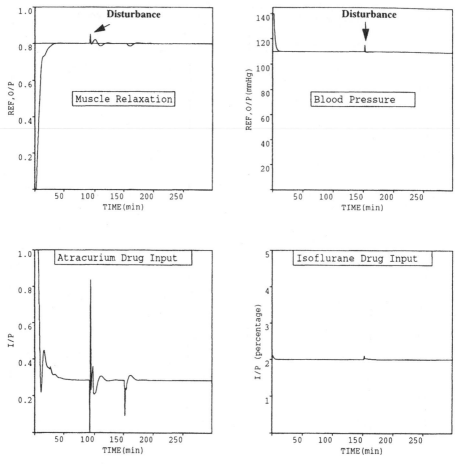

Figure 6.3 Extended GPCF algorithm with $P(z^{-1})$ and $T(z^{-1})$; $N_1 = 1$; $N_2 = 10$; $NU = 1$; $P_1 = P_2 = 2(1 - 0.5z^{-1})$ and $T_1 = T_2 = 1 - 0.9z^{-1}$.

process dynamics and the sampling period. The figure shows that the responses in both channels were well-damped and free from overshoot. It can also be seen that the interaction in the muscle relaxation channel originating from the blood pressure channel was minimised at the cost of overdamping the arterial pressure response.

Phase 2

Phase 2 considered the inclusion of the observer polynomial $T(z^{-1}) = 1 - 0.9z^{-1}$ together with the previous polynomial $P(z^{-1})$ in order to enhance further the robustness of the overall control strategy (Robinson and Clarke, 1991). The same values as before were assumed for N_1, N_2, and NU. Figure 6.2 shows how the effect of disturbances was reduced, but at the same time the output responses were affected because of the use of $P(z^{-1})$. Also the interaction from the blood pressure was reduced. In this result, output disturbances were made during the run being 5% at time 90 minutes in the relaxation dynamics, and 17% (6 mmHg) at time

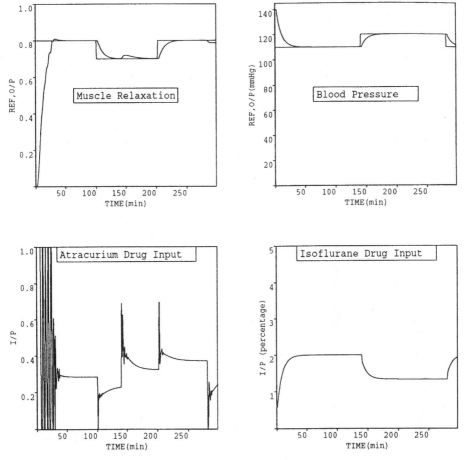

Figure 6.4 Extended multivariable GPC algorithm with $P(z^{-1})$; $N_1 = 1$; $N_2 = 10$; $NU = 2$; $P_1 = P_2 = 10(1 - 0.9z^{-1})$.

150 minutes in the arterial pressure model. Constant set-point command signals of 80% and 110 mmHg for relaxation and blood pressure respectively were considered in this case.

Phase 3

For phase 3 the GPCF algorithm was tuned at the following parameter values:

$$N_1 = 1, \quad N_2 = 10, \quad NU = 1$$

$$T(z^{-1}) = 1 - 0.9z^{-1}$$

$$P(z^{-1}) = \frac{1 - 0.5z^{-1}}{0.5}$$

By introducing the previous disturbances to the system, this run produced the responses of Figure 6.3 where the transients in both channels are seen to be fast and

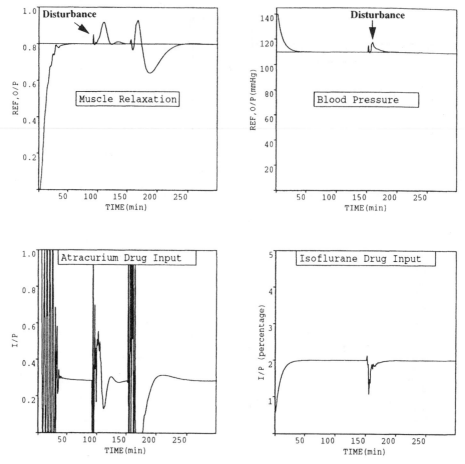

Figure 6.5 Extended multivariable GPC algorithm with $P(z^{-1})$ and $T(z^{-1})$; $N_1 = 1$; $N_2 = 10$; $NU = 2$; $P_1 = P_2 = 10(1 - 0.9z^{-1})$ and $T_1 = T_2 = 1 - 0.9z^{-1}$.

well-damped. The control activity, either during the transient period or later, was low leading to a minimum interaction in the muscle relaxation channel. Again constant set-point commands of 80% and 110 mmHg were used for muscle relaxation and blood pressure respectively.

6.3.2   A comparative study with multivariable GPC using a P-canonical form

It has already been mentioned that an effective alternative for modelling interactions in a multi-loop context is the use of a P-canonical structure for the multivariable model (Kam *et al.*, 1985; Owens, 1981). One direct consequence resulting from this structure is that here too the interactions are introduced in a feedforward manner.

However, as far as estimation is concerned, the A matrices of the $A(z^{-1})$ polynomial are diagonal, whereas the B matrices of the $B(z^{-1})$ polynomial are full rank. In light of these considerations, the same experimental protocol described in Section 4.1 was repeated using the multivariable version of GPC and assuming a

P-canonical structure for the model. Hence, a discrete model of 5 As and 6 Bs with an assumed time delay of 1 sample was considered. All other conditions were similar to those previously outlined.

Figures 6.4, 6.5, and 6.6 show the results of the three runs corresponding respectively to Figures 6.1, 6.2, and 6.3. Figure 6.4 demonstrates similar performance to Figure 6.1 except that in this latter case the control activity was much lower, especially during the transient. Disturbance rejection properties were better in the GPCF case than in the multivariable GPC case where the controller took longer to recover, as Figure 6.5 shows. Finally, Figure 6.6 shows acceptable performance, but that of Figure 6.3 represents a better transient response in the muscle relaxation channel with a moderate control activity which led to a small interaction.

To complement the visual indications of control performance from Figures 6.1 to 6.6, an objective measure of error performance over the simulation runs was made using ISE (integral of squared errors) and ITAE (integral of time and absolute error) criteria. Table 6.1 gives the values for the above figures. The unit of time for the ITAE criterion was minutes. The criteria were evaluated for the 100 minute

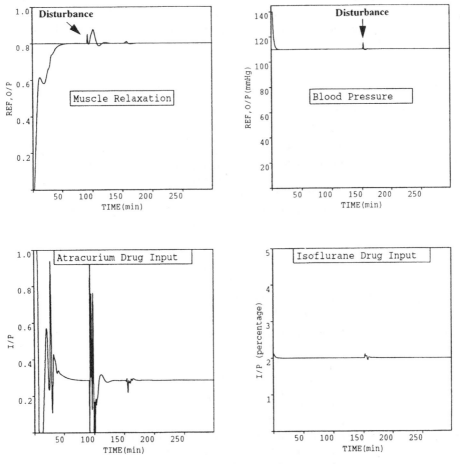

Figure 6.6 Extended multivariable GPC algorithm with $P(z^{-1})$ and $T(z^{-1})$; $N_1 = 1$; $N_2 = 10$; $NU = 1$; $P_1 = P_2 = 2(1 - 0.5z^{-1})$ and $T_1 = T_2 = 1 - 0.9z^{-1}$.

Table 6.1 A comparative table for the different ISE and ITAE criteria corresponding to multivariable GPCF and GPC algorithms

Figure number	Time phases (*min*) from … to …	Paralysis channel		Blood pressure channel	
		ISE	ITAE	ISE	ITAE
6.1	0 to 99	5.16	76	5101	2326
	100 to 200	0.07	179	566	14492
	201 to 300	0.07	274	559	24953
6.2	0 to 300	4.84	182	5127	3771
6.3	0 to 300	3.13	98	2292	1947
6.4	0 to 99	5.17	74	5096	2315
	100 to 200	0.07	176	567	14491
	201 to 300	0.06	272	559	24951
6.5	0 to 300	5.89	1420	5395	14592
6.6	0 to 300	3.81	193	2288	1902

stretches for each set-point change and 300 minutes in the case of a constant set-point. The table indicates comparable values for Figures 6.1 and 6.4 but significantly lower values for channels 1 and 2 for Figures 6.2 and 6.3 than those obtained for Figures 6.5 and 6.6.

Table 6.2 Table representing the speed of execution for different settings of the multivariable GPCF and GPC algorithms

Speed performance relating to GPC: 5 hour simulation run

Figure number	Type of algorithm	Execution time (s)
6.1	Multivariable GPCF algorithm with: $P(z^{-1})$; $N_1 = 1$; $N_2 = 10$; $NU = 2$; $P_1 = P_2 = 10(1 - 0.9z^{-1})$	50.68
6.2	Multivariable GPCF algorithm with: $P(z^{-1})$ and $T(z^{-1})$; $N_1 = 1$; $N_2 = 10$; $NU = 2$; $T_1 = T_2 = 1 - 0.9z^{-1}$; $P_1 = P_2 = 10(1 - 0.9z^{-1})$	51.06
6.3	Multivariable GPCF algorithm with: $P(z^{-1})$ and $T(z^{-1})$; $N_1 = 1$; $N_2 = 10$; $NU = 1$; $T_1 = T_2 = 1 - 0.9z^{-1}$; $P_1 = P_2 = 2(1 - 0.5z^{-1})$	42.68
6.4	Extended multivariable GPC algorithm with: $P(z^{-1})$; $N_1 = 1$; $N_2 = 10$; $NU = 2$; $P_1 = P_2 = 10(1 - 0.9z^{-1})$	123.22
6.5	Extended multivariable GPC algorithm with: $P(z^{-1})$ and $T(z^{-1})$; $N_1 = 1$; $N_2 = 10$; $NU = 2$; $T_1 = T_2 = 1 - 0.9z^{-1}$; $P_1 = P_2 = 10(1 - 0.9z^{-1})$	131.50
6.6	Extended multivariable GPC algorithm with: $P(z^{-1})$ and $T(z^{-1})$; $N_1 = 1$; $N_2 = 10$; $NU = 1$; $T_1 = T_2 = 1 - 0.9z^{-1}$; $P_1 = P_2 = 2(1 - 0.5z^{-1})$	113.94

Finally, an execution time evaluation of the GPCF algorithm and the multi-variable GPC was conducted for the six experiments. Running on a SUN 4 computer, the study produced Table 6.2 showing the different execution times in seconds for a five-hour simulation run. As illustrated in this table, the use of the GPCF algorithm reduced the execution time by a factor of almost 3, hence making the GPCF scheme faster despite the choice of a control horizon greater than 1 in some cases.

6.4   Conclusions

Interactions have always represented the major problem in designing a good controller for a multivariable process. In adaptive control, among the well-known solutions to counteract this interaction problem, the use of a P-canonical structure of the discrete model has been suggested. This has the effect of considering the interactions in a feedforward manner rather than feedback. In this study, another approach is proposed in which the overall multivariable model is seen as two single loops with the interactions modelled as external disturbances via feedforward signals. The algorithm, referred to throughout as GPCF, is shown to be simple to formulate and easy to understand as the whole concept is equivalent to the well-known GPC strategy as outlined by Clarke et al. (1987a, 1987b). One limitation for the application of such a scheme is that the respective delays in the direct paths have to be smaller or equal to the respective delays in the interaction paths. This assumption is reasonable since the process should react first to the major input then to the disturbance. Simulation results using a derived nonlinear model for anaesthesia have shown that the GPCF algorithm is as good as the multivariable GPC for regulation and is better in terms of transient responses, control activity, handling of interactions, and speed.

Moreover, it is known that the use of a $T(z^{-1})$ polynomial can have several advantages (Shook et al., 1991) such as eliminating possible offsets in the data, attenuating high frequency components amplified by Δ, and most importantly reducing the closed-loop feedback gain (see Chapter 3). In a SISO context the choice of $T(z^{-1})$ follows simple guidelines similar to those outlined by McIntosh et al. (1989) and Robinson and Clarke (1991). However, in a multivariable case the choice is more difficult (Mohtadi et al., 1992), and this may be better dealt with if independent single loops are used, linked by feedforward to overcome interaction as is the case with GPCF. A similar scheme has already been validated during real-time experiments on a heat exchanger pilot plant as well as a coupled electric drive pilot plant (Lee et al., 1991) which were both modelled as full-rank systems as opposed to the anaesthesia model which has been modelled as a triangular system (one interactive path only). However, in order to validate further the robustness of the approach clinical trials would be necessary in a similar manner to that already done for SISO GPC of muscle relaxation.

CHAPTER SEVEN

Generalised Predictive Control with Long Range Predictive Identification (LRPI) for Multivariable Anaesthesia

7.1 Introduction

In order to update its model parameters GPC makes use of the recursive least-squares (RLS) identification scheme or any of its variants. Other than the applications reported in this book, many successful applications have been widely reported in many areas of industrial and life sciences whether with SISO GPC or its multivariable version, e.g. cement mills (Al-Assaf, 1988), robot manipulators (Lambert, 1987a), dryers (Lambert, 1987b), tracking systems (Favier, 1987). One common feature of all the above applications lies in the fact that the use of RLS identification in conjunction with GPC was adopted. The parameter estimation issue, however, has wider repercussions on the effectiveness of such an approach. If one wishes to elaborate the problem it is necessary to analyse the model upon which the GPC strategy is based.

Let us recall the model upon which GPC's foundation is laid:

$$A(z^{-1})y(t) = B(z^{-1})u(t-1) + x(t) \tag{7.1}$$

where $y(t)$ is the measured variable, $u(t)$ the control input and $x(t)$ represents the disturbance upon which the model is based and is considered to be of moving average form, i.e.:

$$x(t) = C(z^{-1})\frac{\xi(t)}{\Delta} \tag{7.2}$$

where

$$C(z^{-1}) = c_0 + c_1 z^{-1} + c_2 z^{-2} + \ldots + c_p z^{-p}$$

$\xi(t)$ = an uncorrelated random sequence

$$\Delta = 1 - z^{-1}$$

Substituting equation (7.2) into equation (7.1) and appending the operator Δ leads to:

$$A(z^{-1})\Delta y(t) = B(z^{-1})\Delta u(t-1) + C(z^{-1})\xi(t) \tag{7.3}$$

Equation (7.3) suggests that the data are normally filtered by the operator Δ before being fed to the RLS estimator, and this simple operation can be effective in dealing with offset possibly present in the data. It can, however, be detrimental in an environment dominated by noise due to the properties of Δ which has high-pass characteristics. Parts of the problem were later alleviated by introducing a filter with low-pass characteristics capable of offsetting the effect of Δ at high frequencies. In this case the overall obtained filter will be of the form:

$$\frac{\Delta}{T(z^{-1})}$$

Although the scheme can be incorporated with almost all self-tuning adaptive controllers, its uniqueness in the GPC case lies in the fact that it is included in the control calculations as well. By so doing, this filter plays two important roles, namely:

1. It reduces high frequency components and removes offset possibly present in the input and output data.
2. It attenuates the effect of unmodelled dynamics normally apparent in the high frequency regions and therefore reduces the overall feedback control gain.

Straightforward though this filter idea is, another problem associated with it has to be overcome, namely the choice of its order and its cut-off frequency. Ideally, $T(z^{-1}) = C(z^{-1})$, but since it is practically impossible to estimate the noise polynomial $C(z^{-1})$, the intuitive suggestion that the $T(z^{-1})$ parameters should be equivalent to those of the $\hat{A}(z^{-1})$ polynomial was soon followed by others. Thus, Robinson and Clarke (1991) introduced the notion of stability bound, the bound having to be kept as high as possible to ensure robustness, for which slow observer roots were found to satisfy this requirement. Another idea advanced by McIntosh *et al.* (1989) proposed using different filter characteristics for the controller and the estimator. Recently, the use of positional data for the RLS estimator together with GPC was successfully applied in the operating theatre to regulate the muscle relaxation level by means of continuous drug infusion (see Chapter 2). Amid these successful attempts to alleviate the Δ operator drawbacks, research work conducted by Shook *et al.* (1991, 1992) focused on the idea that the predictions used by the controller strategy should be made equivalent to those used by the identification criterion. The overall identification strategy named long range predictive identification (LRPI) was successfully applied to a real-time SISO control system (Shook *et al.*, 1992) and this chapter reviews the same algorithm when applied to the nonlinear multivariable anaesthetic model previously derived (see Chapter 4) in conjunction with generalised predictive control with feedforward (GPCF) (see Chapter 6) and multivariable GPC using a P-canonical form for the process model (see Chapters 4 and 6). The work is organised into four sections: Section 7.2 briefly reviews the development of the LRPI algorithm and its implementation through filtering, and Section 7.3 describes the simulation studies conducted using GPCF and multivariable GPC. Finally, conclusions regarding the effectiveness of the algorithm are drawn in Section 7.4.

7.2 Development of the long range predictive identification (LRPI) algorithm and its implementation through filtering

7.2.1 Control objective

The GPC cost function at time t is given by the following expression:

$$J_{GPC} = \sum_{j=N_1}^{N_2} [\omega - \hat{y}(t+j/t)]^2 \tag{7.4}$$

where ω is the set-point and $\hat{y}(t+j/t)$ is the prediction of $y(t+j)$ based on information available at time t. Moreover, $\hat{y}(t+j/t)$ represents the best estimate of the future value of the controlled variable y, in other terms, once N_1 and N_2 are specified the controller considers a window of length no bigger than $N_2 - N_1 + 1$.

Consider now a function of GPC which takes into account the control quality as opposed to the predicted control quality of equation (7.4), i.e.:

$$J_{AC} = \sum_{j=N_1}^{N_2} [\omega - y(t+j/t)]^2 \tag{7.5}$$

but

$$y(t+j) = \hat{y}(t+j/t) + \varepsilon_j(t) \tag{7.6}$$

therefore

$$J_{AC} = \sum_{j=N_1}^{N_2} [(\omega - \hat{y}(t+j/t)) - \varepsilon_j(t))]^2 \tag{7.7}$$

or

$$J_{AC} = \sum_{j=N_1}^{N_2} [\omega - \hat{y}(t+j/t)]^2 + \sum_{j=N_1}^{N_2} (\varepsilon_j(t))^2 - 2\sum_{j=N_1}^{N_2} [\omega - \hat{y}(t+j/t)](\varepsilon_j(t)) \tag{7.8}$$

where $\varepsilon_j(t) = y(t+j) - \hat{y}(t+j/t)$ is the j-step ahead prediction error.

The first term of equation (7.8) corresponds to the cost function at time t as in equation (7.4). GPC minimises the value of this term for a given model. The second term is the identification objective, i.e.:

$$J_{ID} = \sum_{j=N_1}^{N_2} (\varepsilon_j(t))^2 = \sum_{j=N_1}^{N_2} [y(t+j) - \hat{y}(t+j/t)]^2 \tag{7.9}$$

Hence, the *optimal* identification method for the control objective of equation (7.5) must provide the model that predicts best, i.e. N_2 steps ahead, unlike the least-squares (LS) method which uses only one step ahead predictions. Equation (7.9) represents the corner-stone of the LRPI philosophy. As for the third term of equation (7.8), it is a term that combines the effect of errors in identification and control and is ignored in all *certainty equivalent control* (Lu and Fisher, 1992).

7.2.2 Formulation of the LRPI algorithm

In order to formulate the steps involved in the LRPI algorithm, it is necessary to draw attention to the analogies that exist between LRPI and the least-squares (LS) formulations. As pointed out earlier, the identification objective is to minimise the value of the second term in equation (7.8). The cost function minimised by LRPI is chosen as the following expression:

$$J_{LRPI} = \frac{1}{t - N_2} \sum_{j=1}^{t-N_2} \frac{1}{N_p} \sum_{j=N_1}^{N_2} [y(k+j) - \hat{y}(k+j/k)]^2 \tag{7.10}$$

where $N_p = N_2 - N_1 + 1$.

It is evident that expression (7.9) is an extension of the standard least-squares regression objective given by the following expression:

$$J_{LS} = \frac{1}{t} \sum_{k=1}^{t} [y(k+1) - \hat{y}(k+1/k)]^2 \tag{7.11}$$

The minimisation of equation (7.10) gives:

$$\frac{\partial J_{LRPI}}{\partial \hat{\theta}} = 0 \tag{7.12}$$

i.e.:

$$\frac{1}{t - N_2} \sum_{k=1}^{t-N_2} \frac{1}{N_p} \sum_{j=N_1}^{N_2} (\hat{y}(t/t - j) - y(t)) \frac{\partial \hat{y}(t/t - j)}{\partial \hat{\theta}} = 0 \tag{7.13}$$

It has been shown that equation (7.13) can be solved using the Newton or Gauss–Newton approach (Shook *et al.*, 1991), but for on-line implementation, where a recursive form of the above algorithm is necessary, the method has been found to be computationally demanding with poor or unknown convergence properties. Instead, the following alternative algorithm has been proposed.

The process is assumed to be of the form:

$$y(t) = \frac{B^0(z^{-1})}{A^0(z^{-1})} u(t - 1) \tag{7.14}$$

The process model is assumed to have the following form:

$$\hat{A}(z^{-1})y(t) = \hat{B}(z^{-1})u(t - 1) + \frac{T(z^{-1})\zeta(t)}{\Delta} \tag{7.15}$$

The noise model:

$$\frac{T(z^{-1})\zeta(t)}{\Delta}$$

is imposed by GPC. The j-step ahead GPC predictor is given by the following:

$$\begin{cases} \hat{y}(t+j/t) = \dfrac{F_j}{T} y(t) + \dfrac{E_j \hat{B}}{T} \Delta u(t+j-1) \\ T = E_j A\Delta + z^{-j} F_j \end{cases} \tag{7.16}$$

The LRPI cost function can be written in terms of the GPC predictor as follows:

$$J_{LRPI} = \frac{1}{t - N_2} \sum_{k=1}^{t-N_2} \frac{1}{N_p} \sum_{j=N_1}^{N_2} \left\{ y(k+j) - \left[\frac{F_j y(k)}{T} + \frac{E_j \hat{B}}{T} \Delta u(k+j-1) \right] \right\}^2 \tag{7.17}$$

using

$$E_j \frac{A\Delta}{T} = 1 - z^{-j} \frac{F_j}{T}$$

and

$$y(k + j) = \frac{B_0}{A_0} u(t - 1)$$

it follows that:

$$J_{\text{LRPI}} = \frac{1}{t - N_2} \sum_{k=1}^{t-N_2} \frac{1}{N_p} \sum_{j=N_1}^{N_2} \left\{ \frac{E_j \hat{A} \Delta}{T} \left[\frac{B^0}{A^0} - \frac{\hat{B}}{\hat{A}} \right] u(k + j - 1) \right\}^2 \tag{7.18}$$

but, the one-step ahead prediction cost becomes:

$$J_{\text{LS}} = \frac{1}{t} \sum_{k=1}^{t} \left\{ \frac{\hat{A} \Delta}{T} \left[\frac{B^0}{A^0} - \frac{\hat{B}}{\hat{A}} \right] u(k - 1) \right\}^2 \tag{7.19}$$

It can be seen that the noise model is included in both expressions (7.18) and (7.19). If an additional filter $L(z^{-1})$ were to be used for identification (Ljung, 1987), the least-squares cost function would be of the following form:

$$J_{\text{LS}} = \frac{1}{t} \sum_{k=1}^{t} \left\{ \frac{L \hat{A} \Delta}{T} \left[\frac{B^0}{A^0} - \frac{\hat{B}}{\hat{A}} \right] u(k - 1) \right\}^2 \tag{7.20}$$

Using the frequency domain, expressions (7.20) and (7.18) become respectively:

$$J_{\text{LS}} = \frac{h}{2\pi} \int_{-\pi/h}^{\pi/h} \left| \frac{L \hat{A} \Delta}{T} \right|^2 \left| \frac{B^0}{A^0} - \frac{\hat{B}}{\hat{A}} \right|^2 \Phi_u(\omega) \, d\omega$$

$$J_{\text{LRPI}} = \frac{h}{2\pi} \int_{-\pi/h}^{\pi/h} \frac{1}{N_p} \sum_{j=N_1}^{N_2} \left| \frac{E_j \hat{A} \Delta}{T} \right|^2 \left| \frac{B^0}{A^0} - \frac{\hat{B}}{\hat{A}} \right|^2 \Phi_u(\omega) \, d\omega \tag{7.21}$$

Comparing the two expressions in (7.21) leads to:

$$|L(\omega)|^2 = \frac{1}{N_p} \sum_{j=N_1}^{N_2} |E(\omega)|^2 \tag{7.22}$$

or

$$L(z^{-1})L(z) = \frac{1}{N_p} \sum_{j=N_1}^{N_2} E(z^{-1})E(z) \tag{7.23}$$

In this case the total filtering action is equivalent to an overall filter of the form:

$$H(z^{-1}) = \frac{L(z^{-1})\Delta}{T(z^{-1})}$$

$$\Delta = 1 - z^{-1}$$

$$T(z^{-1}) = t_0 + t_1 + \ldots + t_t z^{-t} \tag{7.24}$$

$$L(z^{-1}) = l_0 + l_1 z^{-1} + \ldots + l_{N_2-1} z^{-N_2+1}$$

This implies, therefore, that there is more filtering for the parameter estimation than for the control. Figure 7.1 represents the final configuration for implementing GPC with the LRPI-based estimation concept and Figure 7.2 represents the same scheme but modified to include a multivariable structure suitable for anaesthesia control. In this particular case the filter $L(z^{-1})$ would be equivalent to the following diagonal

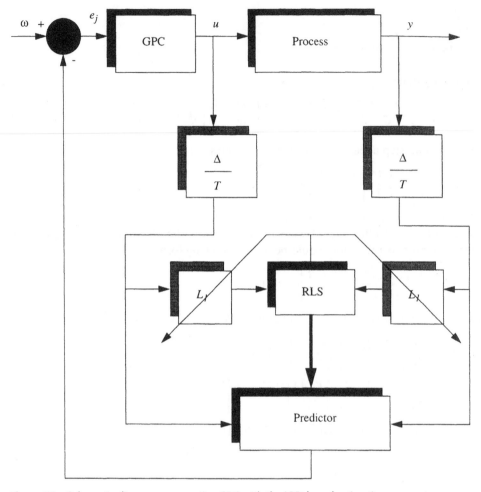

Figure 7.1   Schematic diagram representing GPC with the LRPI-based estimation concept.

filter matrix:

$$L(z^{-1}) = \begin{bmatrix} L_{11}(z^{-1}) & 0 \\ 0 & L_{22}(z^{-1}) \end{bmatrix}$$

This configuration can be justified easily by the fact that in the GPCF case the multivariable system is seen as two SISO loops with feedforward for the interaction, whereas in the multivariable GPC version combined with a P-canonical form for the process model the $A(z^{-1})$ matrix is diagonal, therefore so is the $E(z^{-1})$ matrix.

7.2.3   Properties of the $L_{ii}(z^{-1})$ ($i = 1, 2$) filter

1. If N_1 and N_2 are the chosen horizons, then there is a unique L_{ii} of order $(N_2 - N_1 + 1)$ which satisfies the criterion of equation (7.23).
2. $L_{ii}(z^{-1})$ is a strong function of the output horizon N_2 rather than of the process model, in other words changes in $A(z^{-1})$ are unlikely to affect $L_{ii}(z^{-1})$ very much.

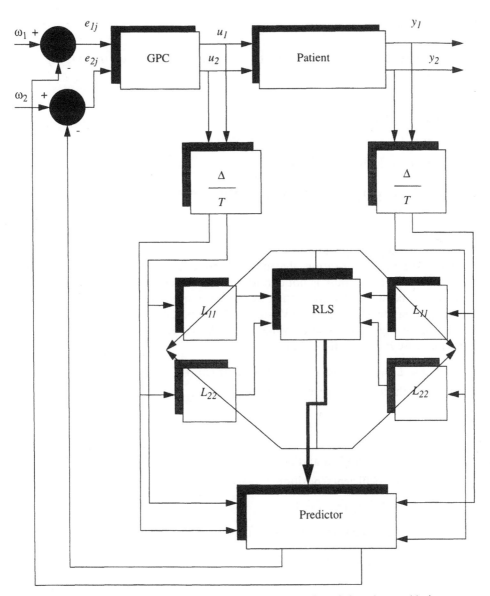

Figure 7.2 Schematic diagram representing GPC with the LRPI-based algorithm modified to enhance a multivariable structure.

3. At each stage of the LRPI algorithm sequence the polynomial $L_{ii}(z^{-1})$, obtained using the spectral factorisation of:

$$\frac{1}{N_p} \sum_{j=N_1}^{N_2} E_{ii}(z^{-1})E_{ii}(z)$$

is **guaranteed stable** although it may not be the spectral factor of the previous sum (this being the key feature of the method).

7.2.4   Computational considerations

The following considerations relate to the implementation of the $L(z^{-1})$ filter. Assume that:

$$
\begin{cases}
E_{ii}(z^{-1}) = e_{i0} + e_{i1}z^{-1} + \ldots + e_{i(N_2-1)}z^{-N_2+1} \\
E_{ii}(z) = e_{i0} + e_{i1}z + \ldots + e_{i(N_2-1)}z^{N_2-1} \\
i = 1, 2
\end{cases}
\tag{7.25}
$$

Using equation (7.23) it follows that:

$$
M_{ii}(z^{-1}) = L_{ii}(z^{-1})L_{ii}(z) = \frac{1}{N_p} \sum_{j=N_1}^{N_2} E_{ii}(z^{-1})E_{ii}(z)
\tag{7.26}
$$

$$i = 1, 2$$

Implemented recursively, the solution of equation (7.26) follows the steps included in Peterka's spectral factorisation algorithm (Bohm *et al.*, 1984). The case where the $A(z^{-1})$ matrix is of full rank is not considered here, where it is believed that another variant of spectral factorisation such as the Newton gradient algorithm would be more appropriate (Kucera and Vostry, 1976) especially since the multivariable version of the algorithm is also available (Jezek and Kucera, 1986). Hence, in this particular case Peterka's algorithm is as follows:

1. Initialise $L_{ii} = 1$ (or to a particular filter structure if known *a priori*).
2. Perform the following deconvolution operation:

    $$
    Q_{ii} = z^{-N_2+1} \frac{M_{ii}(z^{-1})}{L_{ii}(z^{-1})} + \frac{Rem_{ii}}{L_{ii}(z^{-1})}
    $$

    where Q_{ii} is the quotient and Rem_{ii} is the remainder $i = 1, 2$.
3. Reorder the coefficients' positions:

    $$
    Q1_{ii} = z^{-N_2+1}Q_{ii}(z) \quad i = 1, 2
    $$

4. Divide the $Q1_{ii}$ coefficients by the first coefficient:

    $$
    Q2_{ii}(z^{-1}) = \frac{Q1_{ii}(z^{-1})}{q1_{i0}} \quad i = 1, 2
    $$

5. GOTO 2 until convergence.
6. If convergence, then perform the following operation which ensures that the filter gain is unity:

    $$
    L_{ii}(z^{-1}) = \frac{Q2_{ii}(z^{-1})}{\sum\limits_{m=0}^{N_2-1} q2_{im}} \quad \text{for } i = 1, 2
    $$

As seen from the steps above, the algorithm requires successive polynomial divisions (deconvolutions), and in a self-tuning mode the polynomial $M_{ii}(z^{-1})$ is reconstructed every sample because of the changing $E_{ii}(z^{-1})$, but $L_{ii}(z^{-1})$ is retained from the iteration of the previous sample. It is also worth noting that convergence in this case is tested by checking that the norm of the remainder polynomial $Rem_{ii}(z^{-1})$

does not exceed a certain prespecified threshold or tolerance value, i.e.:

IF:

$$Rem_{ii}(z^{-1}) = rm_{i0} + rm_{i1}z^{-1} + \ldots + rm_{i(nrem-1)}z^{(1-nrem)} \quad \text{for } i = 1, 2$$

THEN:

$$\text{Norm}(Rem_{ii}(z^{-1})) = \sum_{m=0}^{nrem-1} |rm_{im}| \leq \text{tolerance} \tag{7.27}$$

However, usually up to three iterations within one sample of control are sufficient, since convergence is quite rapid.

7.3 Simulation results

The simulation studies considered the nonlinear multivariable model for anaesthesia derived in Chapter 4. For parameter estimation, a UD factorisation method was used on incremental data with initial covariance matrix and forgetting factor given by: $Cov = 10^2 . I$ and $\rho = 0.975$. In the multivariable GPC case, a multivariable model of 5 diagonal $A(z^{-1})$ matrices together with 5 upper triangular $B(z^{-1})$ matrices was estimated (see Chapter 4). In the GPCF case, however, a third-order model with a time delay of 1 minute and with two coefficients for the feedforward was considered for the first channel (muscle relaxation), while for the second channel (blood pressure) a first-order model also with a 1 minute time delay was considered (see Chapter 6).

Initial conditions were 0% relaxation and 100 mmHg arterial pressure. The set-point command signal was 80% then 70% for relaxation, and 80 mmHg then 70 mmHg for the blood pressure. A bolus dose u_1 of atracurium of 67 mg at 1 mg ml^{-1} concentration was applied initially for one sample and input u_2 was kept at 0. While the bolus effect took place, the loop remained open until the output in the muscle relaxation channel reached the safety level of 85% when the loop was closed. The self-tuner was allowed to run with the initial parameter estimates until sample time 39 min (where the information vector gathers reasonable data) at which time the parameter estimation routine was allowed to be operational. In all the experiments, which were conducted over a fixed period time of 900 minutes, output disturbances of 6% and 7 mmHg at sample times 70 min and 170 min in the muscle relaxation and the blood pressure channels respectively were applied. These harsh conditions will test the robustness of the GPCF and multivariable GPC strategies combined with both schemes, i.e. RLS and LRPI with respect to their ability to reject the previous disturbances more effectively.

The study was divided into two parts: the first part concerned the application of the GPCF algorithm, whereas the second part considered the multivariable version of GPC together with a P-canonical form of the process model. For each case two identification modes were considered: RLS using an *ad hoc* filter (which is incidentally included in the control law), and LRPI together with the same filter (the idea of more filtering for estimation than control is included here). The $L(z^{-1})$ coefficients, for both channels, were initially taken to be 0.0 except the first one which was taken to be 1.0, and the LRPI sequence was triggered 10 samples after the RLS was switched on. At each sample time the spectral factorisation was carried out with a tolerance of 0.001. The above experiments were conducted in noise-free and noise-

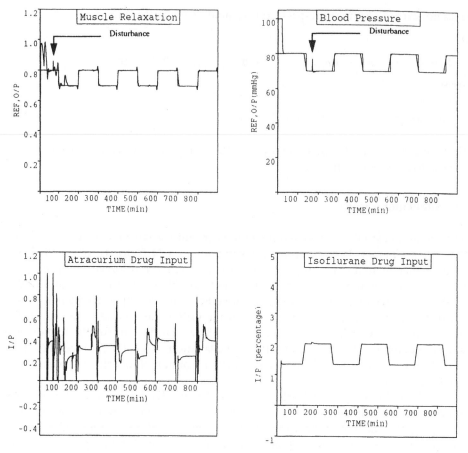

Figure 7.3   Adaptive control of the anaesthetic model; noise-free case; GPCF + RLS + ad hoc $T(z^{-1})$.

contaminated environments. In the latter case, noise sequences of 1% and 5 mmHg peak for the muscle relaxation channel and the blood pressure channel were considered respectively. In either case the adopted GPC tuning knobs were as follows:

$N_1 = 1$

$N_2(\text{ch } 1) = 10$

$N_2(\text{ch } 2) = 15$

$NU(\text{ch } 1) = 2$

$NU(\text{ch } 2) = 1$

$P = I$

and

$$T(z^{-1}) = \begin{bmatrix} (1 - 0.8z^{-1})^2 & 0 \\ 0 & (1 - 0.8z^{-1})^2 \end{bmatrix}$$

for control and estimation.

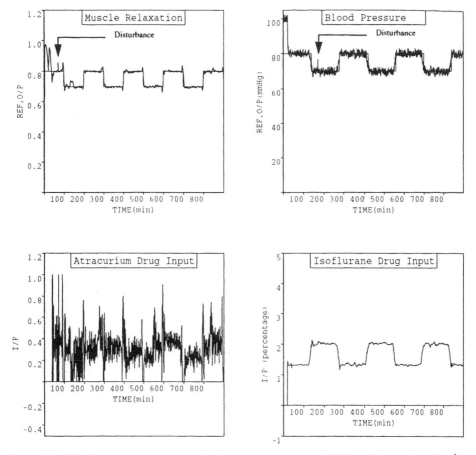

Figure 7.4   Adaptive control of the anaesthetic model; noisy case; GPCF + RLS + ad hoc $T(z^{-1})$.

At this stage it is also worth noting that the set-point profile was pre-specified to the GPC algorithm N_2 samples in advance, this having the effect of reducing the interaction in the muscle relaxation loop (this concept of set-point pre-specification will be discussed fully in Chapter 9).

7.3.1   GPCF with RLS-based identification

For the GPCF algorithm together with the RLS and the *ad hoc* filter $T(z^{-1})$, the simulations produced the output responses of Figures 7.3 and 7.4 in a noise-free and noise-contaminated environment respectively. Although the interactions from the second channel were reduced to low levels in both cases, it can also be seen that in Figure 7.3 the disturbance rejection property was not totally adequate due to the fact that the parameter estimates were greatly disturbed.

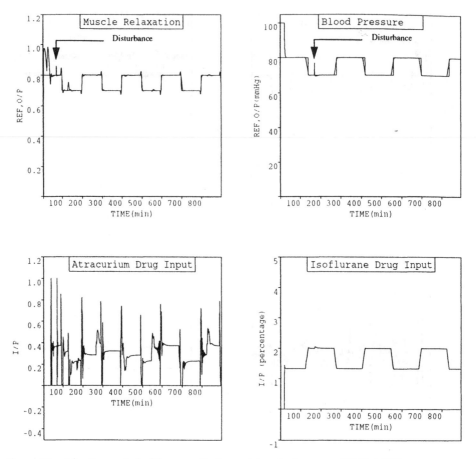

Figure 7.5 Adaptive control of the anaesthetic model; noise-free case; GPCF + LRPI.

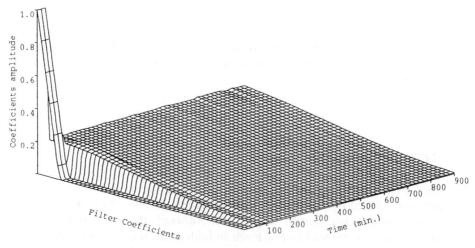

Figure 7.6 Three-dimensional representation of the $L_{11}(z^{-1})$ coefficients for the experiment of Figure 7.5, channel 1.

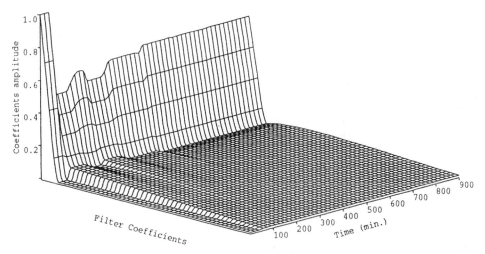

Figure 7.7 Three-dimensional representation of the $L_{22}(z^{-1})$ coefficients for the experiment of Figure 7.5, channel 2.

7.3.2   GPCF with LRPI-based identification

The same experiments were repeated with GPCF being combined with the LRPI-based estimation scheme. The performance of Figure 7.5 was obtained for the noise-free case and it clearly demonstrates that the output disturbance at time 70 min in the relaxation channel was dealt with more effectively than in the RLS case (see Figure 7.3). Figures 7.6 and 7.7 represent the variations of the filters coefficients (in both channels respectively) using a three-dimensional perspective, thus confirming property (2) of Section 7.2.3 namely that the changes in $A(z^{-1})$ do not affect

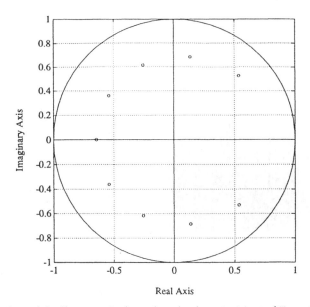

Figure 7.8 Locations of the filter roots in the z-plane for the experiment of Figure 7.5, channel 1.

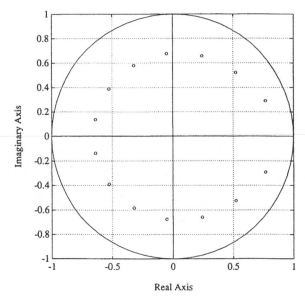

Figure 7.9   Locations of the filter roots in the z-plane for the experiment of Figure 7.5, channel 2.

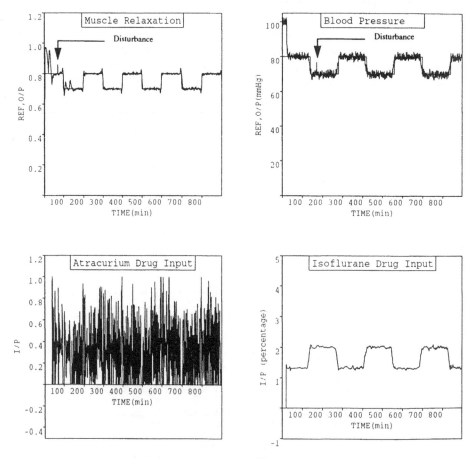

Figure 7.10   Adaptive control of the anaesthetic model; noisy case; GPCF + LRPI.

$L(z^{-1})$ very much. In turn, Figures 7.8 and 7.9 show the locations of the filter zeros in the z-plane and confirm property (3) of Section 7.2.3, namely that the filter structure is stable.

Figures 7.10, 7.11 and 7.12 represent the equivalent of the above case but with the outputs corrupted with randomly generated noise. It can be seen that the input signal to the muscle relaxation channel was highly activated in contrast to a reasonably active signal in the second channel, this latter being relatively easier to control

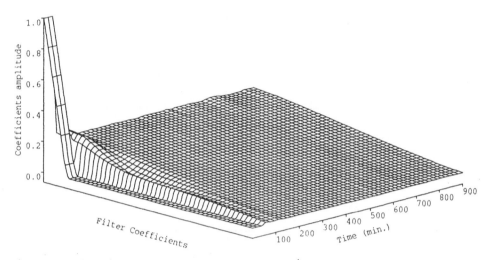

Figure 7.11   Three-dimensional representation of the $L_{11}(z^{-1})$ coefficients for the experiment of Figure 7.10, channel 1.

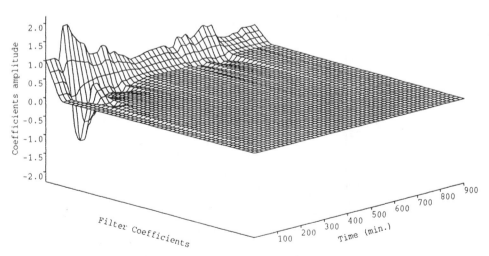

Figure 7.12   Three-dimensional representation of the $L_{22}(z^{-1})$ coefficients for the experiment of Figure 7.10, channel 2.

since it involves a simple first-order system with no interaction from the other channel.

The high control activity in the muscle relaxation channel however, can be explained by the fact that the value of the control horizon 'NU' was higher than 1 and also that the structure of $L(z^{-1})$ was amplifying the variations originating from the blood pressure channel. Figures 7.13 and 7.14 display the locations of the filter zeros in the z-plane indicating stability. In fact, further investigations into the loca-

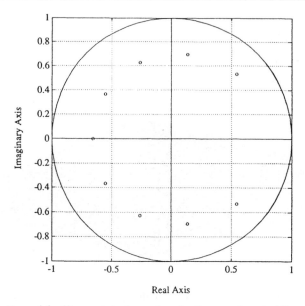

Figure 7.13   Locations of the filter roots in the z-plane for the experiment of Figure 7.10, channel 1.

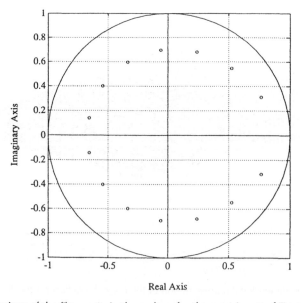

Figure 7.14   Locations of the filter roots in the z-plane for the experiment of Figure 7.10, channel 2.

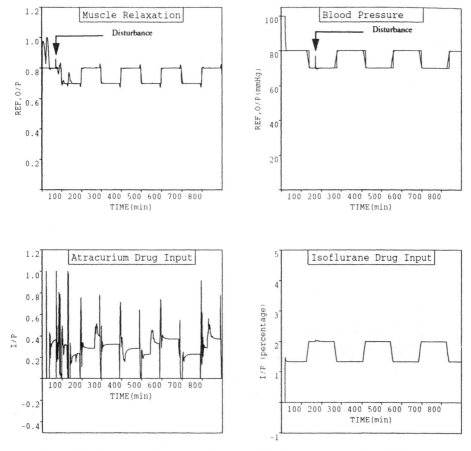

Figure 7.15   Adaptive control of the anaesthetic model; noise-free case; multivariable
GPC + RLS + ad hoc $T(z^{-1})$.

tion of the filter roots suggested the presence of fast characteristics which are not favoured in a highly stochastic case. It should be noted, however, that the output variances in both channels were better minimised under such a scheme.

7.3.3   Multivariable GPC with RLS-based identification

If the multivariable structure of GPC is used under the same conditions as above, the resulting performances can be compared with those for the trials with GPCF. With the RLS-based estimation concept the performances were those of Figures 7.15 and 7.16 respectively for noise-free and noise-contaminated environments. Here too the interactions were kept small despite the absence of the $P(z^{-1})$ polynomial, but the reaction to the disturbance in the first channel followed the same trend as in the GPCF case.

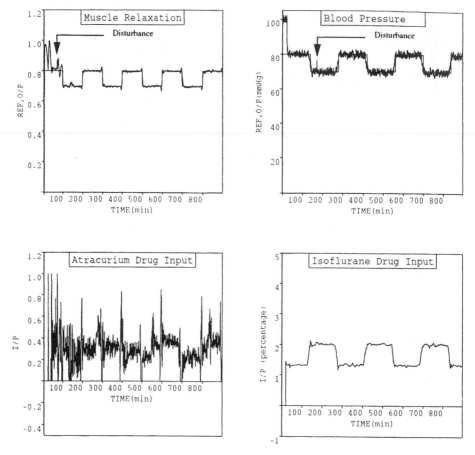

Figure 7.16 Adaptive control of the anaesthetic model; noisy case; multivariable GPC + RLS + ad hoc $T(z^{-1})$.

7.3.4 Multivariable GPC with LRPI-based identification

With the LRPI-based estimation technique, according to Figure 7.17, the reaction to the disturbance was better despite the fact that the output value just before the disturbance was below its target. Figures 7.18 and 7.19 represent the evolution of the filters' coefficients for the 900 minute run, the first of which indicates that they scarcely settled during the first 100 samples. Also, Figures 7.20 and 7.21 show the locations of the filter zeros which demonstrate filter stability. Another feature of this trial is the sudden filter variations from time 615 min which caused the control signal in the first channel to violate its constraints and this in turn led to an output overshoot. Although these variations cannot be considered as severe, it is worth emphasising that since the parameters are still estimated by a standard RLS scheme only using data filtered by an extra filter it is advisable to adopt extra measures which would prevent 'bursting' or 'blow-up' phenomena such as covariance reset-ting, variable forgetting factor and/or perturbation signals. Indeed, when noise was

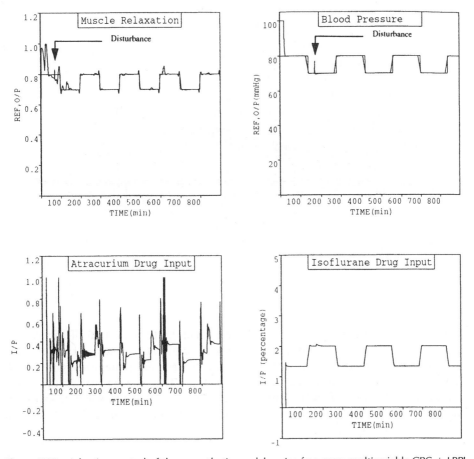

Figure 7.17 Adaptive control of the anaesthetic model; noise-free case; multivariable GPC + LRPI.

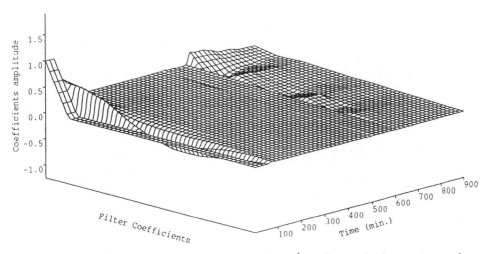

Figure 7.18 Three-dimensional representation of the $L_{11}(z^{-1})$ coefficients for the experiment of Figure 7.17, channel 1.

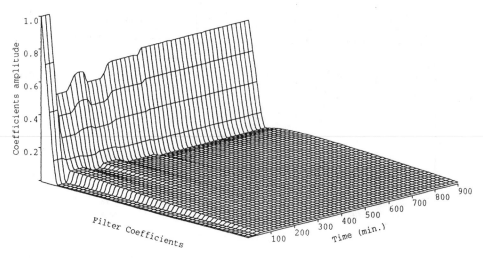

Figure 7.19   Three-dimensional representation of the $L_{22}(z^{-1})$ coefficients for the experiment of Figure 7.17, channel 2.

included, the performance of Figure 7.22 was much better than that of Figure 7.17 as far as the output variance and the disturbance properties in the first channel were concerned, but similarly to the GPCF case the control still remained highly active. Figures 7.23 and 7.24 show the variations of the filters' coefficients for the whole run. Figure 7.23 indicates better and more settled characteristics when proper excitation was provided for the estimation. Figures 7.25 and 7.26 show the locations of the filter zeros in the z-plane.

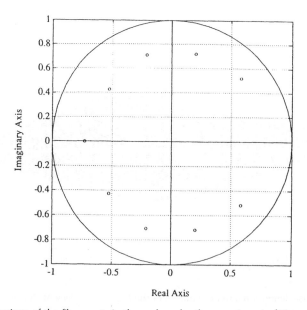

Figure 7.20   Locations of the filter roots in the z-plane for the experiment of Figure 7.17, channel 1.

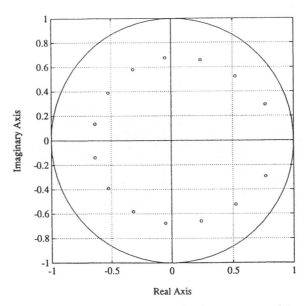

Figure 7.21 Locations of the filter roots in the *z*-plane for the experiment of Figure 7.17, channel 2.

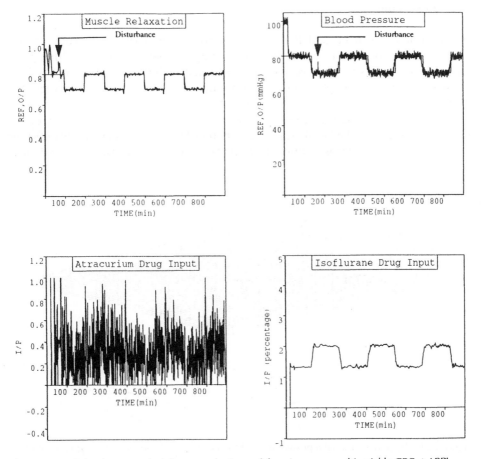

Figure 7.22 Adaptive control of the anaesthetic model; noisy case; multivariable GPC + LRPI.

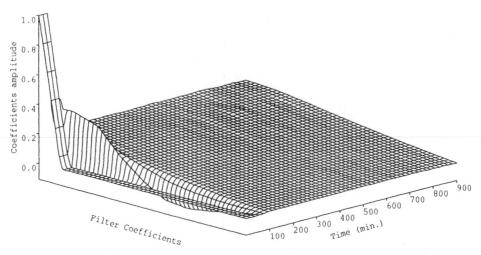

Figure 7.23   Three-dimensional representation of the $L_{11}(z^{-1})$ coefficients for the experiment of Figure 7.22, channel 1.

7.4   Conclusions

In conclusion, it can be said that the LRPI concept is a very interesting scheme since it takes into account the predictions used by the GPC algorithm. Although its formulation might suggest a very complicated and difficult algorithm, it has been modified to be much simpler and to incorporate better convergence properties. The result is the use of more filtering for the estimation than for control by adding a regressor filter whose structure depends more on the output horizon N_2 than on the process poles. In fact the key feature in computing $L(z^{-1})$ is **the spectral factorisation** which is a series of deconvolution operations easily realised even in an adaptive

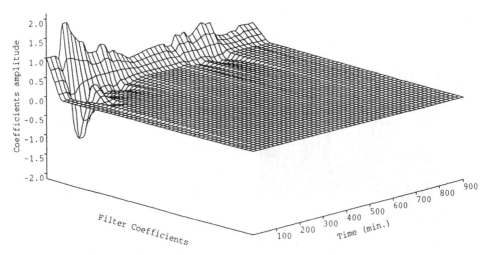

Figure 7.24   Three-dimensional representation of the $L_{22}(z^{-1})$ coefficients for the experiment of Figure 7.22, channel 2.

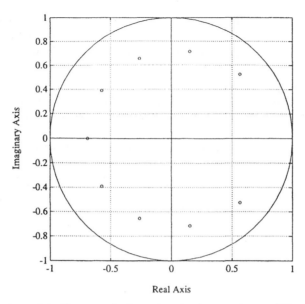

Figure 7.25 Locations of the filter roots in the *z*-plane for the experiment of Figure 7.22, channel 1.

manner. Successfully applied by its original authors to a SISO control system, this chapter considered its application to a multivariable structure where the inter-actions are considered in a feedforward manner. Simulations on a difficult nonlinear multivariable anaesthetic model using two control strategies, i.e. GPCF and multi-variable GPC with a P-canonical structure, showed that under the LRPI scheme the GPC algorithm was able to reject the disturbances more effectively than the RLS

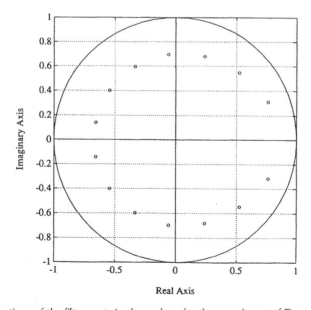

Figure 7.26 Locations of the filter roots in the *z*-plane for the experiment of Figure 7.22, channel 2.

scheme. Also, the role of the $L(z^{-1})$ filter as a 'deterrent' against process mismatch could be seen for the GPCF case. For instance, the estimated feedforward terms were limited to two, whereas normally more are estimated. Moreover, it can also be seen from the different trials that the output variance is minimised better under the LRPI scheme than it is under RLS. However, when high noise levels are superimposed on the outputs, the control activity seems to be amplified by the whole filter structure. Yoon and Clarke (1994) have already discussed this problem which they associate with the wrong choice of the $T(z^{-1})$ polynomial order with respect to that of the $A(z^{-1})$ polynomial in the model. For this particular application and from an engineering point of view, if one is not so concerned about the levels of interaction, then perhaps a low value of the control horizon (i.e., $NU = 1$) would be more appropriate in this case.

CHAPTER EIGHT

A Comparative Study between Multivariable Generalised Predictive Control and Intelligent Self-organising Fuzzy Logic Control (SOFLC) for Multivariable Anaesthesia

8.1 Introduction

In recent years, much attention has been given in control systems research and development to algorithms which have learning properties. Two common branches in a taxonomy of learning algorithms comprise *self-adaptive* systems (e.g. self-tuning control) and *self-organising* systems. In both cases, one is concerned with the control of systems with unknown or time-varying structure or parameters. The purpose of this chapter is to explore these two forms of learning control in the area of biomedicine where structural uncertainty is the rule rather than the exception.

In contrast to the theory of self-tuning adaptive control already introduced in the beginning of this book, another area which has seen growing interest among control engineers is that of intelligent control. It, like the former technique, had to wait until significant development had occurred in computer technology before its associated algorithms could be implemented. Indeed, for many years it has been the scientists' dream to be able to duplicate as faithfully as possible a human's behaviour simply by using computers. One consequence of this, as far as feedback control systems are concerned, is that if the designed control strategy bears similarities to that of a human brain, the control could in some sense be optimal. Fuzzy control is one qualitative strategy that endeavours to do that, and originates in the theory of fuzzy logic, first introduced by Zadeh (1965, 1973). The theory has proved to be partly successful in representing fuzziness in human decision-making behaviour. From a structural point of view the controller is represented by a set of rules built via guidelines normally provided by an experienced operator well aware of the process under investigation. Consequently, the controller looks at the process as a black box and does not need an accurate model description. Following some successful applications of fuzzy control in automation by pioneers such as Assilian and Mamdani (1974), the so-called Self-Organising Fuzzy Logic Controller (SOFLC) was later introduced by Procyk (1977). The algorithm is able to realise adaptation by building its fuzzy rules on-line as it controls the process, altering and adding as many rules as it judges necessary from off-line criteria. This approach has seen several successful applications (Daley and Gill, 1986; Linkens and Mahfouf, 1988; Harris and Moore, 1989; Linkens and Hasnain, 1991) and it is suggested that it represents a serious contender to quantitative approaches for control.

Hitherto, little work has been reported apart from Al-Assaf (1988) in which the two approaches, different perhaps in their concept but having the same aim, are experimentally compared, and in which disadvantages as well as advantages of both strategies are discussed. The experimental area is that of control of anaesthetic drug administration in the operating theatre.

To investigate the performance associated with the two approaches of multivariable self-tuning adaptive GPC and multivariable SOFLC, we have considered the possibility of simultaneous control of relaxation and unconsciousness during anaesthesia (see Chapter 4). Although the model presented here is well-defined structurally, it should be noted that in reality there is considerable uncertainty attached to it. The model does, however, offer a realistic multivariable challenge to the two approaches, particularly because of the severe nonlinearity in the relaxant pharmacodynamics. Following a brief review of the multivariable SOFLC in Section 8.2, a series of comparative simulation results follow in Section 8.3, with concluding remarks from the study in Section 8.4.

8.2   Review of multivariable self-organising control using fuzzy logic

8.2.1   Description of a simple fuzzy controller

Fuzzy set theory and approximate reasoning were introduced by Zadeh (1965, 1973), and its general idea is to incorporate the concept of fuzzy linguistic variables as a means of describing qualitative relationships. The fuzzy variables, therefore, allow rigorous statements to be made about approximate quantities and appear to offer a method of having both uncertainty in the description of a process and intuition about the way it should be controlled. For instance, conventional theory teaches us that there is a difference between elements which belong to a set and those which do not. For example, if one wants to specify linguistic measurement of temperature on a closed interval (100–200 °C), then for a temperature greater than or equal to 150 °C, an ordinary set which defines this can be expressed in terms of membership to this set by a membership function μ which takes values of either 0 (when the temperature is not a member of the set) or 1 (when the temperature is a member of the set). A similar fuzzy set might be defined as 'Temperature much greater than 150 °C' or 'Temperature about 150 °C'. In both cases the membership function takes values between the interval (0, 1) which would indicate the degree of membership to the set.

Various mathematical operators have been assigned to the theory of fuzzy set (Zadeh, 1965, 1973) which make its analysis possible. Such operators can be found in the literature but perhaps the most important one is **the composition rule of inference** operator '∘' which is defined as follows.

To infer the output U from given process state E, CE and fuzzy relation R, the compositional rule of inference gives:

$$U = CE \circ (E \circ R) \tag{8.1}$$

Although the theory of fuzzy sets originated in the mid-sixties, it was only in the mid-seventies that fuzzy logic control, which is based on fuzzy logic, was given an engineering thrust by Mamdani (Assilian and Mamdani, 1974; King and Mamdani, 1977) who implemented the first fuzzy logic controller on a boiler and steam engine, and this opened a wider door to more applications in various fields of industry and the life sciences.

A simple rule-based fuzzy logic controller is designed to regulate the output of a process around a given set-point, the output of the process being sampled at a regular interval and sent to the controller. Figure 8.1 shows the configuration of the simple fuzzy control scheme. There are two inputs to the controller, the error (E) which is the difference between the process output and the reference target and the change in error (CE) which is simply its derivative. The output from the controller is (U) which is also the process input. The overall control rules which regulate the process can be represented as in Table 8.1. A typical rule should read:

If error (E) is 'Big' and

change in error (CE) is 'Small'

then output (U) is 'Big'

The sequence of calculations in a simple fuzzy logic control (FLC) scheme is as follows.

First, and referring to Figure 8.1, error (E) and change in error (CE) are calculated according to the above given definitions, and the variables being representatives of crisp values are fuzzified after being scaled. Next, and according to the rules supplied from the rule-based block, the fuzzy control is inferred then converted into a crisp value by a defuzzification procedure before being scaled and sent to the process. It is worth noting that in such configurations the **fuzzy rule-base** contains a set of rules whose number and definitions are fixed (they need not be) during the whole run. However, the controller can be given an adaptive role by modifying the same rules (the number of the contributing rules can be made to change together with the definition of each rule); hence the controller is known as a self-organising fuzzy logic control (SOFLC) scheme as shown in the next section.

8.2.2 The self-organising fuzzy logic control (SOFLC) algorithm

As illustrated in Figure 8.2 the self-organising fuzzy logic controller (SOFLC) comprises two main levels. The first level consists of a simple fuzzy controller, whereas the second acts as a monitor and a performance evaluator of the previous level and is usually called the self-organising mechanism. It includes four blocks: the performance index, the process reference model, the rules modifier, and the state buffer.

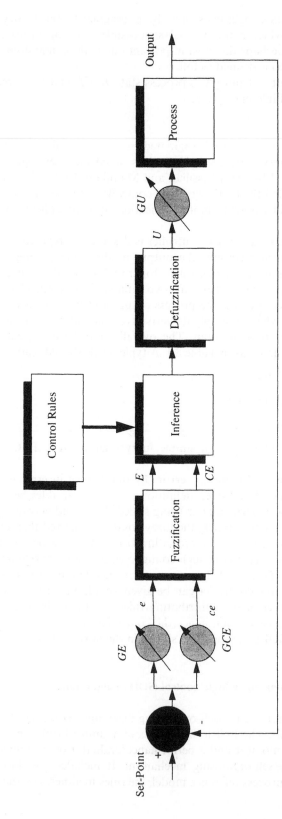

Figure 8.1 Block diagram of a simple fuzzy logic control (FLC) scheme.

Table 8.1   A simple fuzzy rule-based table

	CE		
E	Small	Zero	Big
Small	Small		Big [Controller output (U)]
Zero	Small	Zero	
Big	Big		

In the first level, the input signal to the controller is taken at each sampling instant in the form of error and change in error. Each signal is mapped to its correspondent discrete level by using the error and change in error scaling factors respectively, and sent to the SOFLC. According to the control rules issued by the second level the SOFLC calculates the outputs with respect to the inputs. The output signals are scaled to actual values using the output scaling factors and afterwards sent to the process being controlled.

The first level is a simple fuzzy logic controller, containing a set of control rules. The latter are derived from linguistic expressions and interpreted by fuzzy logic (King and Mamdani, 1977). Many parameters affect the design of this crucial part such as: the **fuzzification** procedure, the choice of the input and output variables, the type of fuzzy control rules, the implication and **inference** procedure, as well as the **defuzzification** operation. In this work, the fuzzy sets associated with the input and the output variables were formed upon discrete **universes of discourse** of 14, 13, and 15 elements respectively for error, change in error, and output. The choice of the membership function forming a particular fuzzy set is based on Mizumoto's findings (Mizumoto, 1988) that the fuzzy sets are best selected when the **fuzzy labels** are not isolated and not overlapped too much. Therefore, the linguistic labels are the same as those reported previously in other studies, where the terms PO and NO respectively define values slightly below zero. They were mainly introduced to obtain finer control around the equilibrium state. The control rules are linguistic conditional statements, symbolised in the form of a relational matrix R, with the fuzzy output being obtained using Zadeh's compositional rule of inference (Zadeh, 1973; Harris and Moore, 1989). Several procedures allow one to reduce this fuzzy set to a single value, via defuzzification. Among these methods are the mean of maxima (MOM) procedure (Assilian and Mamdani, 1974), and the centroid of area method (COA) (Harris and Moore, 1989). Because the latter allows for smoother variations in the control signal, it was adopted in these studies.

The second level is basically the part that realises the adaptation referred to above. Based on observations of the trajectory of the process being controlled, any deviation from the desired path is corrected by modifying the rules responsible for that particular undesirable deviation.

The performance index function is an evaluation criterion of the controller performance, and is derived from linguistic conditional statements using standard fuzzy operations as shown in Table 8.2. The entries in this table have the usual fuzzy linguistic connotation of N = Negative, P = Positive, O = Zero, B = Big, S = Small, and M = Medium. The rule modification procedure can be explained as follows. Assuming that the process has a time delay of m samples, then the control action at sample $(nT - mT)$ has most contributed to the process performance at the

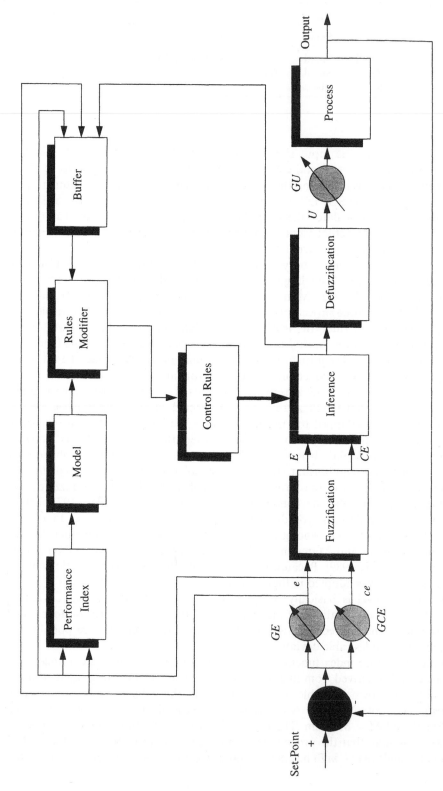

Figure 8.2 Block diagram of a self-organising fuzzy logic control (SOFLC) scheme.

Table 8.2   The performance index table

Error	Change in error						
	NB	NM	NS	ZO	PS	PM	PB
NB	NB	NB	NB	NM	NM	NS	ZO
NM	NB	NB	NM	NM	NS	ZO	PS
NS	NB	NB	NS	NS	ZO	PS	PM
NO	NB	NM	NS	ZO	ZO	PM	PM
PO	NB	NM	ZO	ZO	PS	PM	PB
PS	NM	NS	ZO	PS	PS	PB	PB
PM	NS	ZO	PS	PM	PM	PB	PB
PB	ZO	PS	PM	PM	PB	PB	PB

sampling instant nT, thus the modification is made to the controller output mT samples earlier, and therefore the rule to be included will be:

$$E(nT - mT) \rightarrow CE(nT - mT) \rightarrow U(nT - mT) + P_i(nT) \qquad (8.2)$$

where $P_i(nT)$ is issued by the performance index. To avoid contradictory rules, only rules with similar antecedents to the new rule must be removed. An algorithm for rules removal was presented (Daley and Gill, 1986) which can be expressed linguistically as:

Delete all the rules that are the same ones as to be added

The process reference model relates the input changes to the output changes, and can be derived simply by considering a two-input two-output process characterising a general state-space equation (Procyk and Mamdani, 1979). For small changes in the inputs, one can write:

$$\begin{bmatrix} \Delta X \\ \Delta Y \end{bmatrix} = \begin{bmatrix} T \, \partial \dot{X} \\ T \, \partial \dot{Y} \end{bmatrix} = M \begin{bmatrix} \Delta U \\ \Delta V \end{bmatrix} \qquad (8.3)$$

where M is regarded as an incremental model of the process. Therefore, if the performance index outputs are $P_{i1}(nT)$ and $P_{i2}(nT)$, then the necessary input corrections $P_{o1}(nT)$ and $P_{o2}(nT)$ are given by:

$$\begin{bmatrix} P_{i1}(nT) \\ P_{i2}(nT) \end{bmatrix} = M^{-1} \begin{bmatrix} P_{o1}(nT) \\ P_{o2}(nT) \end{bmatrix} \qquad (8.4)$$

where

$$M = \begin{bmatrix} m_{11} & m_{12} \\ m_{21} & m_{22} \end{bmatrix}$$

The model M should be scaled from real values to normalised values using scaling factors for each variable, details of which follow. Thus,

$$P_i(nT) = (GT)^{-1}(M)^{-1}(GY)^{-1}P_o(nT) \qquad (8.5)$$

(where GT and GY are scaling factors) P_o should not exceed the maximum or the minimum range defined initially. The condition is therefore satisfied if:

$$(S_1)^{-1} = \frac{m_{11}}{GY_1 GT_1} + \frac{m_{12}}{GY_1 GT_2} \leq 1$$

$$(S_2)^{-1} = \frac{m_{21}}{GY_2 GT_1} + \frac{m_{22}}{GY_2 GT_2} \leq 1$$

(8.6)

This yields:

$$M = \text{scale}(GT)^{-1}(M)^{-1}(GY)^{-1}$$

(8.7)

where

$$\text{scale} = \min[S_1, S_2]$$

The state buffer is a FIFO (first in, first out) register which records the values of the error and change in error, as well as the output. The output from the register will be recorded after a time equal to the delay-in-reward. This latter parameter plays a vital role in modifying the rules, since it specifies which input in the past contributed to the present performance. It is suggested that a value equal to the dead-time of the process is appropriate (Procyk, 1977).

8.2.3 Selection of the controller parameters

As mentioned before, the different variables used are scaled before entering the algorithm, and the selection of the respective scaling factors is not entirely subjective since their magnitude is a compromise between the sensitivity during the transient period and the required steady state accuracy. Useful guidelines leading to the choice of these parameters are given below, and these were used in initial tuning of the simulation results which follow.

The error scaling factor was chosen according to the percentage value and is given by the following:

$$GE = \frac{6.0}{\text{full error}}$$

$$\text{full error} = \text{error percentage} \times \text{set-point}$$

(8.8)

The value of the error percentage decides the sensitivity of the previous scaling factor. Associated high values mean small scaling factors, while low values imply large ones.

The change in error scaling factor (GCE) was chosen according to the maximum real change in error for each variable giving:

$$GCE = \frac{6.0}{\text{max real error change}}$$

(8.9)

In contrast to the previous ones, the output scaling factor was chosen to accommodate the controller output to the process input according to the following relation:

$$GT = \frac{\text{max process input}}{\text{max controller output}}$$

(8.10)

Further details about recommendations for the selection of these scaling factors can be found in Linkens and Abbod (1992).

8.3   Simulation studies

The simulation studies were undertaken in two parts, the first being concerned with evaluation of both algorithms using nominal process parameters. In each case, the design parameters were refined by extensive simulation studies carried out by one of the authors. The second consisted of selecting the process parameters using a randomised Monte-Carlo approach. For all the continuous models being considered, a fourth-order Runge–Kutta method with fixed step length was used for the numerical integration.

8.3.1   Simulation studies using nominal parameter values

The nonlinear multivariable model described in Chapter 4 was simulated in continuous form. A series of simulations was considered for both algorithms on different machines, the GPC being implemented on a SUN workstation, whereas the SOFLC was run on a single T800 Transputer with a host PC.

The study used a step length of 0.1 and a sampling interval of 1 minute. Initial conditions were 0% relaxation and 140 mmHg arterial pressure. For both algorithms, the set-point command signal was 80% for relaxation, and 110 mmHg for blood pressure.

As well as discussing the performances of both designs, a comparison of the respective execution times is also given.

Performance of the adaptive GPC algorithm

In this case, during the first 25 samples, initial control was provided by the self-tuner but with fixed parameter estimates obtained from the nominal linear model. The input signal was clipped between 0 and 1.0 for the atracurium drug input, and between 0% and 5% for the isoflurane input. A further maximum limit of 0.5 was placed on the atracurium input during the initial 25 samples (where the parameter estimates were fixed) to prevent excessive fluctuations in drug demand. For parameter estimation, a UD-factorisation method (Bierman, 1977) was used on incremental data, with an initial covariance matrix and forgetting factor given by $Cov = 10^2.I$, $\rho = 0.995$ respectively.

A discrete multivariable model with 5 diagonal $A(z^{-1})$ and 6 full-rank $B(z^{-1})$ parameters were estimated with an assumed time delay of one sample. The experiments were conducted in three phases to determine suitable tuning parameter settings.

Phase 1 investigated the basic algorithm, in contrast to phase 2 and 3 which were concerned with the extended algorithm using respectively the model-following polynomial $P(z^{-1})$ and the observer polynomial $T(z^{-1})$. Figure 8.3 shows one result from phase 1 where the controller parameter settings were different between the two

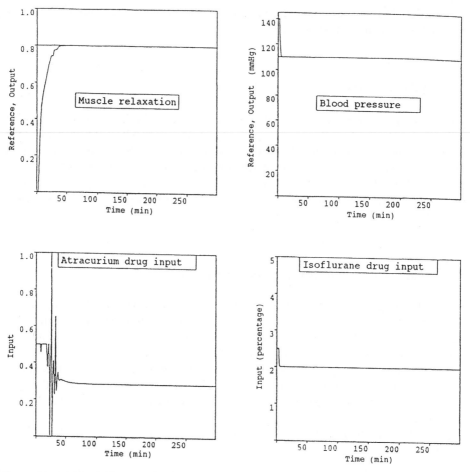

Figure 8.3 Multivariable generalised predictive control (GPC) investigation with differential channel parameters: $N_1 = 1$; $N_2(\text{ch } 1) = 10$; $N_2(\text{ch } 2) = 20$; $NU(\text{ch } 1) = 1$; $NU(\text{ch } 2) = 2$.

channels: $N_1 = 1$, $N_2(\text{ch } 1) = 10$, $N_2(\text{ch } 2) = 20$, $NU(\text{ch } 1) = 1$, $NU(\text{ch } 2) = 2$. This result gave fast responses particularly for arterial pressure.

Phase 2 was concerned with the model-following polynomial $P(z^{-1})$. Based on the particular dynamics as well as the sampling period, a time constant of approximately 10 minutes (identical for both channels) was selected for assignment of the P matrix. Figure 8.4 shows how this could be used to produce a smooth response in the relaxation channel as well as minimising the interaction, at the cost of over-damping in the arterial pressure channel.

Finally, phase 3 considered the inclusion of the important observer polynomial $T(z^{-1})$. Figure 8.5 shows how the effect of disturbances could be reduced without affecting the closed-loop responses. In this result, output changes were made during the run, being 5% at time 90 min in the relaxation dynamics, and 10% (5 mmHg) at time 150 min in the arterial pressure model. From these figures, it can be seen that the control action for atracurium is severe during the initial transient, but this is reduced significantly by inclusion of the observer polynomial.

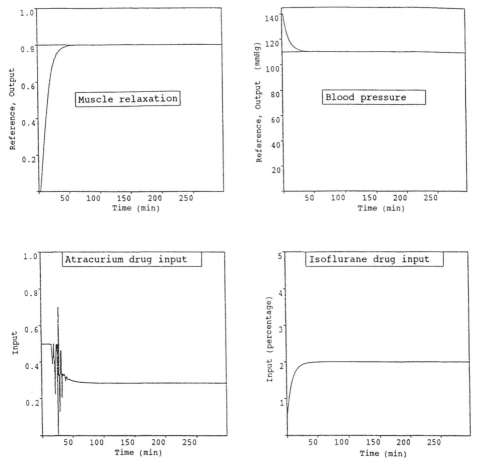

Figure 8.4   Extended multivariable GPC with model-following polynomial $P(z^{-1})$: $N_1 = 1$; $N_2 = 10$; $NU = 2$; $P_1 = P_2 = (1 - 0.9z^{-1})/0.1$.

Performance of the SOFLC algorithm

Under the same conditions as those described in Section 8.3.1, the study considered two versions of the algorithm. The simple version consists of a fixed set of scaling factors, while the extended one includes switching from one set of scaling factors to another. Multi-run tests with a maximum of three runs for each case were conducted starting with an initially empty controller (i.e. no rules). The rules were then stored at the end of each run and used as a starting point for the following one.

Figure 8.6 shows a result where the simple controller was used with the following small scaling factors:

$$GE_1 = 11.36 \quad GCE_1 = 30.0 \quad GT_1 = 0.166 \qquad \text{for channel 1}$$

$$GE_2 = 0.333 \quad GCE_2 = 0.30 \quad GT_2 = 0.45 \qquad \text{for channel 2}$$

With these settings the controller gave a fair control policy for the two channels. In the first run, the output for channel 1 exhibited an undershoot due to the fact that the controller started with no rules at all, whereas the output for channel 2 was fast

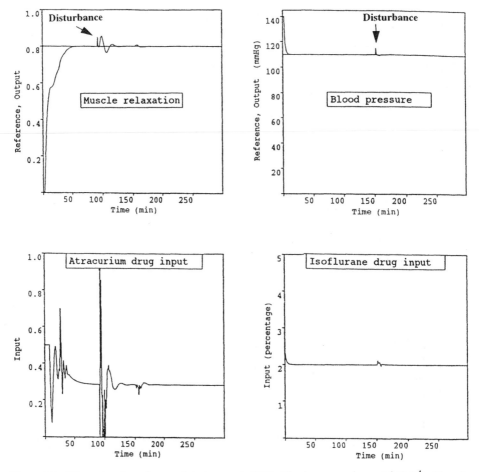

Figure 8.5 Effect of output change disturbances in GPC with observer polynomial $T(z^{-1})$; $N_1 = 1$; $N_2 = 10$; $NU = 2$; $T_1 = T_2 = (1 - 0.9z^{-1})$.

and adequately damped. During the second and third runs, the previous undershoot was removed. The presence of a steady state error for the first channel (muscle relaxation) could be explained by the choice of low scaling factors which scale the error to positive or negative fuzzy labels which suggest that there is no process output error at all. Table 8.3 also summarises the number of rules generated at the end of each run which was on average 22 and 12 respectively for the first and second channels.

Using the same controller, another experiment was conducted but this time using high scaling factors. The following values were adopted:

$GE_1 = 45.18$ $GCE_1 = 35.0$ $GT_1 = 0.166$ for channel 1

$GE_2 = 1.205$ $GCE_2 = 0.45$ $GT_2 = 0.45$ for channel 2

As shown in Figure 8.7, the controller removed the undershoot in the first channel produced during the first run, as well as reducing the steady state error making the controller therefore more accurate. It did, however, produce a highly active control

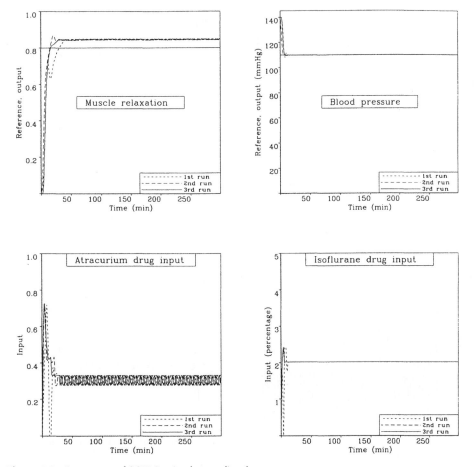

Figure 8.6   Responses of SOFLC using low scaling factors.

signal in the relaxation channel. Also, Table 8.3 shows that the number of rules generated increased to 27 and 22 respectively for the first and second channels due to the higher sensitivity with the chosen scaling factors.

Taking into account the fact that low scaling factors lead to a relatively good transient response on the one hand and a large steady state error on the other, and

Table 8.3   Parameters relating to the simple SOFLC algorithm

| | | | Number of rules | |
Figure	Run	EP (%)	Paralysis	Δ MAP
8.6	1st	66.66	15	10
	2nd	66.66	22	12
	3rd	66.66	22	13
8.7	1st	16.66	18	15
	2nd	16.66	21	20
	3rd	16.66	27	22

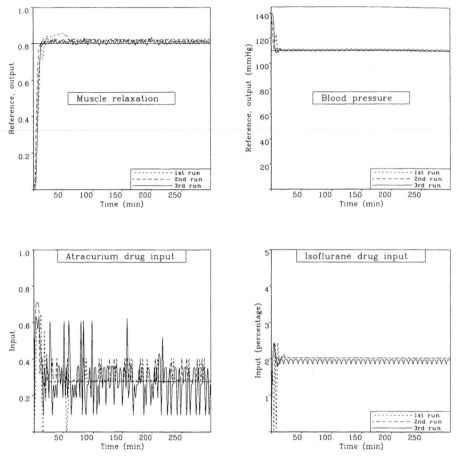

Figure 8.7   Responses of SOFLC using high scaling factors.

that high scaling factors give generally good accuracy in the steady state period but with a larger rule-base size and active control signals, the idea of merging the two techniques seems attractive. This was the object of the third experiment within the framework of an extended controller. To reduce the number of generated rules and also to obtain a good control strategy during the transient response, the controller started with small scaling factors then switched to higher ones. The switch of the scaling factors from one mode to another was programmed in such a way as to occur when the output reached 83% of its final value ($Y_s = 83\%$). Depending on four adopted regimes, the switch could occur on none of the channels, the first channel only, the second channel only, or both channels. Table 8.4 summarises the four regimes.

Extensive simulation studies, beyond the scope of this chapter, showed that regime 3 gave the best performance as far as the size of the rule-base and control signal activity were concerned. Therefore, an experiment was conducted along these lines and whose responses shown in Figure 8.8 demonstrate a good control even during the first run for both channels. These tended to improve even more during

Table 8.4 Table representing the various regimes relating to the extended SOFLC

Regimes	Switch dependent
0	No switch
1	Paralysis channel
2	Δ MAP channel
3	Independent

the second and third runs without an increase in the rule-base size as Table 8.5 illustrates.

Through simulation studies performed on the nominal process model, examples of which have been presented in Section 8.3.1, experience was gained on the selection of the crucial design parameters for GPC and SOFLC. Like many biomedical systems, however, anaesthetic models have very large inter-patient variability for which there is no information prior to an operation. The next section describes the use of the experience gained from the nominal model in the case of randomised model investigations.

8.3.2 Simulation studies via Monte-Carlo parameter selection method

Clearly, the application of these algorithms to this particular multivariable nonlinear anaesthetic model requires many design parameters to be selected, and this selection is very important in a safety critical situation such as an operating theatre. Therefore, in order to validate further the robustness of these control strategies, Monte-Carlo simulations were chosen to undergo such tests. Equation (8.11) describes the model with parameters which are known to vary from patient to patient:

$$\begin{bmatrix} \text{Paralysis} \\ \Delta \text{ MAP} \end{bmatrix} = \begin{bmatrix} \dfrac{K_1(1 + T_4 s)e^{-\tau_1 s}}{(1 + T_1 s)(1 + T_2 s)(1 + T_3 s)} & \dfrac{K_4 e^{-\tau_4 s}}{(1 + T_6 s)(1 + T_7 s)} \\ 0 & \dfrac{K_2 e^{-\tau_2 s}}{(1 + T_5 s)} \end{bmatrix} \begin{bmatrix} U_1 \\ U_2 \end{bmatrix} \quad (8.11)$$

The nonlinearity is still represented by the Hill Equation (2.7) described in Chapter 2 using the same parameters, although these could have been randomised.

Table 8.5 Parameters relating to the extended SOFLC algorithm

Figure	Run	Y_s (%)	Regime	EP (%) Before	EP (%) After	Number of rules Paralysis	Number of rules Δ MAP
8.8	1st	83	3	66.66	16.66	20	12
	2nd	83	3	66.66	16.66	23	16
	3rd	83	3	66.66	16.66	23	18

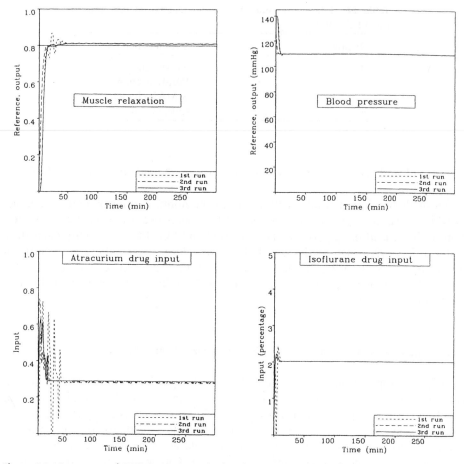

Figure 8.8   Responses of SOFLC using switched scaling factors under regime 3.

The Monte-Carlo simulations consisted of choosing the model parameters in a random manner using the following formula:

$$\text{Monte-Carlo parameter} = \text{Min} + \text{Random} \times (\text{Max} - \text{Min}) \tag{8.12}$$

where $0 < \text{Random} < 1$, and Random is obtained from a random number generator. The Min and Max values for each parameter were chosen to reflect probable pharmacological ranges known to exist. In this way many combinations could be produced. Table 8.6 shows a sample of ten cases which were studied but due to lack of space only three of these will be presented for discussion. Cases 4, 5 and 7 were selected for a comparison of the multivariable GPC and SOFLC algorithms. These cases were chosen to indicate the best, worst and medium performance conditions for each algorithm. The conditions as described in Section 8.3.1 remained unchanged except that the fixed GPC mode was operational only for the first 10 samples and during which the control signal was clipped between 0 and 0.50. For the multivariable SOFLC algorithm, the extended version of regime 3 was adopted using the same scaling as before with the exception of the change in error scaling

Table 8.6 Selected model parameters using Monte-Carlo method

Monte-Carlo simulation method

Anaesthetic model parameters

Case number	T_1	T_2	T_3	T_4	K_1	T_5	K_2	T_6	T_7	K_4
1	2.54	4.17	27.88	14.89	2.01	1.57	−17.26	2.79	1.19	0.24
2	2.45	4.28	16.44	7.30	1.69	1.54	−17.70	3.01	1.33	0.27
3	2.35	5.95	27.88	10.88	2.16	1.15	−14.61	3.06	1.26	0.24
4	1.18	5.10	31.26	10.31	1.34	1.14	−15.94	2.99	1.26	0.24
5	1.36	3.84	32.00	7.31	2.46	1.20	−10.48	2.42	1.25	0.27
6	1.55	2.58	32.74	13.31	2.08	1.26	−15.02	2.85	1.24	0.25
7	1.73	5.32	33.48	10.31	1.71	1.31	−19.55	3.28	1.22	0.27
8	1.91	4.06	34.22	7.31	1.33	1.37	−14.09	2.71	1.21	0.25
9	2.09	2.80	34.96	13.30	2.45	1.43	−18.63	3.14	1.20	0.27
10	2.27	5.54	15.70	10.30	2.07	1.49	−13.61	2.57	1.18	0.25

factors where a compromise set of values suiting most cases had to be found. The adopted values were:

$$GC_1 = 1.0, \quad GCE_2 = 0.10$$

Figure 8.9 shows the performance of the extended version of GPC using case 4 with the model-following polynomial $P(z^{-1})$ having a relatively fast time constant of 1.44 minutes. The responses in both channels were fast and well damped with the overshoot reduced to a low level in channel 1 which exhibits severe nonlinearities.

Case 5 represented a severe test for the chosen GPC configuration, as was also the case for SOFLC. It corresponds to a high gain muscle relaxation model, and a low gain blood pressure model. Figure 8.10 shows a good performance for blood pressure, but a heavy initial overshoot in the relaxation channel and subsequent saturation of drug signals. Finally, case 7 represented a medium condition with inferior blood pressure response to that of Figure 8.8, but similar paralysis behaviour as shown in Figure 8.11.

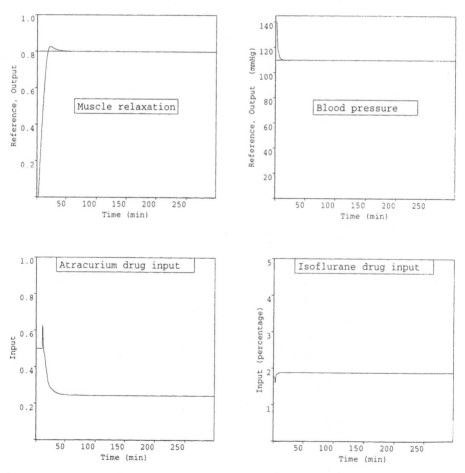

Figure 8.9 Monte-Carlo simulation, case 4: extended multivariable GPC: $N_1 = 1$; $N_2 = 10$; $NU = 1$; $P_1 = P_2 = (1 - 0.5z^{-1})/0.5$.

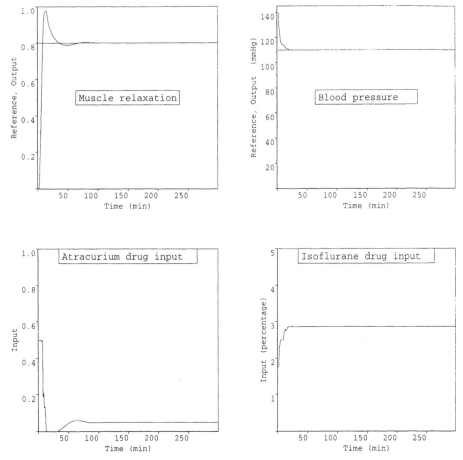

Figure 8.10 Monte-Carlo simulation, case 5: extended multivariable GPC: $N_1 = 1$; $N_2 = 10$; $NU = 1$; $P_1 = P_2 = (1 - 0.5z^{-1})/0.5$.

The next series of experiments considered the SOFLC algorithm. Figure 8.12 illustrates how the controller behaved on the model with the parameters of case 4. The responses in both channels were quite good although the control signals were highly active. The worst performance was recorded when using the model parameters of case 5. The responses shown in Figure 8.13 demonstrated large steady state errors in both channels, mainly because the switch from a set of low scaling factors to a set of high scaling factors did not take place. For case 7 shown in Figure 8.14, the control signals were highly active and led to a limit cycle in channel 1. Table 8.7 summarises the controller parameters and the number of generated rules during the three experiments.

To complement the visual indications of control performance, an objective measure of error performance over the simulation run was made using ISE (integral of squared errors) and ITAE (integral of time and absolute error) criteria. Table 8.8 gives the ISE and ITAE values for GPC and SOFLC respectively for all the Figures 8.3 to 8.14. The unit of time for the ITAE criterion was minutes in each case. The

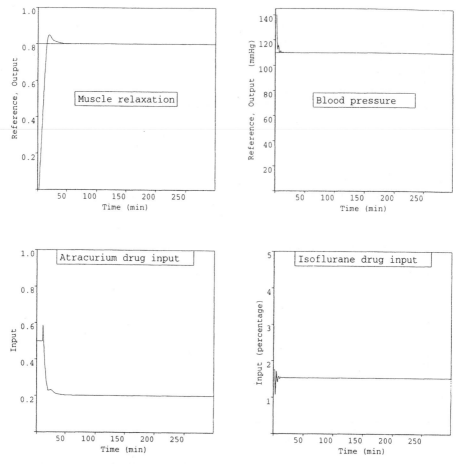

Figure 8.11 Monte-Carlo simulation, case 7: extended multivariable GPC: $N_1 = 1$; $N_2 = 10$; $NU = 1$; $P_1 = P_2 = (1 - 0.5z^{-1})/0.5$.

criteria were evaluated over the whole 300 minute run in each case. This length of run is much longer than the transient settling time, and hence accentuates any steady state error in the ITAE evaluation. This is particularly evident in the SOFLC values.

In general, all the ITAE values were greater than the ISE values, because of the time scale involved. Similarly, all the blood pressure ITAE and ISE values were greater than for paralysis, simply because of the non-normalised values for blood pressure. Approximate normalisation of blood pressure ISE could be obtained via division by 10,000 and ITAE via division by 100. This would give relatively lower figures for blood pressure than paralysis in both GPC and SOFLC. This reflects clearly the better dynamic performance for the simpler linear dynamic of that channel. In Figures 8.3 to 8.8 the GPC and SOFLC parameters were experimentally tuned to obtain a good control performance for the particular design selection and scaling factor choice. This is reflected in the ISE and ITAE entries for these figures,

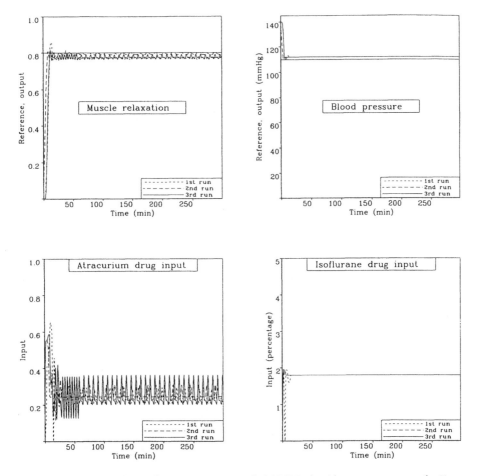

Figure 8.12 Monte-Carlo simulation, case 4: extended SOFLC algorithm; parameters as for Figure 8.7, except that $GCE_1 = 1.0$; $GCE_2 = 0.10$.

where it is seen that there is little difference between the values for Figures 8.3 to 8.5 and Figures 8.6 to 8.8. The well-known sensitivity of ITAE to errors at large time is shown clearly in the case of Figure 8.8. Whereas the ISE for paralysis shows little differential indication between the runs, the ITAE measure for the third run shows a definite degradation in performance. This is also indicated in the blood pressure response, where the large increase in ITAE is hardly evidenced visually in Figure 8.8.

Turning now to the Monte-Carlo results, we can discuss differences in performance between GPC and SOFLC. For case 4 which both algorithms found easy to control, SOFLC gave better ISE for paralysis (indicating a faster initial response), but worse ITAE and ISE for blood pressure. Both GPC and SOFLC found case 5 difficult to manage, which is not surprising because of the extreme nature of the parameters. SOFLC gave large ISE and ITAE because of its inability to reduce steady state errors for either paralysis or blood pressure, this being true for each of

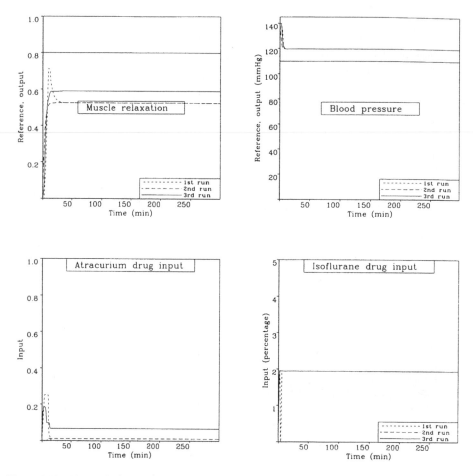

Figure 8.13   Monte-Carlo simulation, case 5: extended SOFLC algorithm; parameters as for Figure 8.7, except that $GCE_1 = 1.0$; $GCE_2 = 0.10$.

the runs. In contrast, GPC provided reasonable control. The third case, selected visually as moderate performance, indicated a better performance by SOFLC in terms of ISE for paralysis, but better blood pressure performance for GPC.

8.3.3   Execution time considerations

An execution time evaluation for both algorithms was conducted for all the previous experiments. For implementation reasons, the algorithms were run on different machines. The multivariable GPC was run on a SUN computer, whereas the multivariable SOFLC used a single T800 transputer. The study produced Tables 8.9 and 8.10 where the corresponding execution times in seconds for each type of algorithm are shown for a standard simulation run of 5 hours. The study suggests that both algorithms would perform adequately here, considering a real-time sampling of 1 minute in this anaesthetic application! It took on average 0.35 seconds for

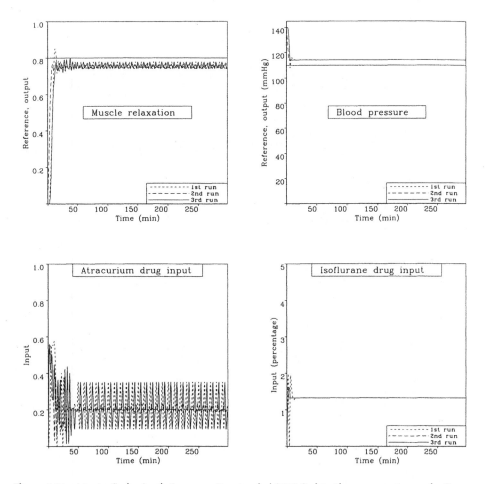

Figure 8.14 Monte-Carlo simulation, case 7: extended SOFLC algorithm; parameters as for Figure 8.7, except that $GCE_1 = 10$; $GCE_2 = 0.10$.

Table 8.7 The fuzzy controller parameters

Figure	Case	Run	Y_s (%)	EP (%) Before	EP (%) After	Number of rules Paralysis	Number of rules Δ MAP
8.12	4	1st	83	66.66	16.66	10	8
		2nd	83	66.66	16.66	13	8
		3rd	83	66.66	16.66	13	8
8.13	5	1st	83	66.66	16.66	5	2
		2nd	83	66.66	16.66	7	2
		3rd	83	66.66	16.66	7	2
8.14	7	1st	83	66.66	16.66	11	8
		2nd	83	66.66	16.66	12	10
		3rd	83	66.66	16.66	12	11

Table 8.8 Table representing the ISE and ITAE criteria for equivalent GPC and SOFLC runs

GPC

Figure number	Paralysis		Δ MAP	
	ISE	ITAE	ISE	ITAE
8.3	3.34	60	2073	84
8.4	5.93	112	5096	2316
8.5	3.91	189	2215	2081
8.9	3.75	42	2126	63
8.10	2.98	60	2707	584
8.11	3.84	43	1979	139

SOFLC

Figure number	Run number	Paralysis		Δ MAP	
		ISE	ITAE	ISE	ITAE
8.6	1st	3.52	307	2435	4151
	2nd	3.34	297	2411	4140
	3rd	3.33	297	2410	4140
8.7	1st	4.65	242	4058	15172
	2nd	3.96	227	3289	15011
	3rd	3.95	227	3285	15008
8.8	1st	3.22	56	2565	7254
	2nd	3.03	94	2427	4631
	3rd	3.95	227	3285	15008
8.12	1st	3.16	226	2943	12699
	2nd	2.89	113	2530	12946
	3rd	3.13	250	2584	11954
8.13	1st	10.5	1488	13510	53503
	2nd	11.7	1561	13510	53503
	3rd	10.1	1442	13510	53503
8.14	1st	3.13	207	2750	11603
	2nd	2.99	205	2935	15862
	3rd	2.91	151	2981	15865

Table 8.9 Table representing the speed of execution for different settings of the multivariable GPC algorithm

Speed performances relating to GPC; 5 hour simulation run		
Figure number	Type of algorithm	Execution time (s)
8.3	Basic multivariable algorithm: $N_1 = 1$; $N_2(\text{ch } 1) = 10$; $N_2(\text{ch } 2) = 20$; $NU(\text{ch } 1) = 1$; $NU(\text{ch } 2) = 2$	124.8
8.4	Extended multivariable algorithm with model-following polynomial $P(z^{-1})$: $N_1 = 1$; $N_2 = 10$; $NU = 2$; $P_1 = P_2 = \dfrac{1 - 0.9z^{-1}}{0.1}$	116.3
8.5	Extended multivariable algorithm with observer polynomial $T(z^{-1})$: $N_1 = 1$; $N_2 = 10$; $NU = 1$; $T_1 = T_2 = 1 - 0.9\ z^{-1}$	94.4
8.9, 8.10 and 8.11	Extended multivariable algorithm with model-following polynomial $P(z^{-1})$: $N_1 = 1$; $N_2 = 10$; $NU = 1$; $P_1 = P_2 = \dfrac{1 - 0.9z^{-1}}{0.1}$	99.4

the GPC to finish one iteration for calculations, whereas 0.033 seconds was needed for the SOFLC execution. The SOFLC formulation was considerably faster than the GPC algorithm, but the use of a transputer constitutes a big advantage over a normal processor. A previous study using SOFLC has, in fact, shown a ten-fold increase in speed by using a transputer-based system against a SUN 3 workstation (Linkens and Hasnain, 1991). In this case, a single T800 transputer was also used, albeit in a slightly different hardware configuration. It is, however, worth noting that the choice of controller parameters is crucial not only for the final performance but also for the computer burden. For instance, in the case of GPC, larger N_2, NU,

Table 8.10 Table representing the speed of execution for different versions of SOFLC

Speed performances relating to SOFLC; 5 hour simulation run				
Figure number	Type of algorithm	Execution time (s)		
		1st run	2nd run	3rd run
8.6	Simple controller: low scaling factors	2.8	3.1	3.1
8.7	Simple controller: high scaling factors	2.8	3.1	3.2
8.8	Extended controller: regime 3	3.6	3.8	4.0
8.12	SOFLC with switch mode	3.2	3.6	3.7
8.13	SOFLC with switch mode	2.2	2.4	2.3
8.14	SOFLC with switch mode	3.2	3.6	3.7

etc., give bigger matrix calculations. In the case of SOFLC, the size of the rule-base produced by modifying, deleting and adding rules is directly influenced by the choice of the performance model as well as the scaling factors for the error, change in error and the output.

8.4   Discussions and conclusions

The multivariable anaesthetic model represents a challenging and realistic basis on which to compare control strategies. The system dynamics are of moderate complexity, but more importantly they contain significant and pharmacologically valid nonlinearities. Of particular relevance, however, is the large patient-to-patient variability in model parameters. This is well-known phenomenon in the life sciences, where parameter variations of 4:1 are endemic, known examples being in muscle relaxation (Linkens *et al.*, 1982) and blood pressure (Slate, 1980). It was because of oscillations observed in some operations performed using parameter PID control strategies that advanced adaptive methods have been introduced. Thus, pole-placement self-tuning was applied to muscle relaxation (Linkens *et al.*, 1985), while a mixed switching controller with Smith prediction for delay compensation, together with gain adaptation, was introduced for blood pressure control (Slate, 1980).

The examples cited above for self-adaptive control refer to SISO systems. Similarly, self-organising approaches have been studied for biomedicine. Fuzzy logic control for biomedicine is attractive, since it offers the possibility of good control without the knowledge of a detailed mathematical model of the process. The problem of rule elicitation is obviated using SOFLC. For muscle relaxation it has been shown that SOFLC can perform well, even with large model mismatches and with an initially empty knowledge base (Linkens and Hasnain, 1991). Similarly, the GPC algorithm used in the current studies has been evaluated in the SISO and MIMO cases, both via simulation and clinical trials (see Chapter 2).

For the multivariable anaesthesia problem the GPC algorithm has been refined via extensive simulations (see Chapter 4). Suitable settings of the many design parameters for the application of GPC were obtained via these studies and previous SISO experience, and have been used in this comparative study. They represent a serious attempt to obtain the best performance via this control strategy. The major design feature of SOFLC is the settings of the scaling factors. Considerable experience has been gained in heuristic methods for selecting these scaling factors via a number of SISO and MIMO laboratory-based engineering rigs (Linkens and Abbod, 1991). Again, this knowledge has been used to obtain the best performance of the same pharmacological process via SOFLC. It remains then to discuss the relative performance between serious attempts at optimised control using the two different approaches.

In general, the GPC results show a smoother performance both in the individually adjusted examples of Figures 8.3 to 8.5 and in the Monte-Carlo runs of Figures 8.9 to 8.11. The control of paralysis is considerably harder than for control of unconsciousness. This is partly due to differences in linear pharmacokinetics, but is mainly caused by the severely nonlinear pharmacodynamics of relaxation. To obtain smooth control action, however, it was necessary to perform many trials using the model-following and observer polynomials of the extended form of GPC (see Figures 8.3 to 8.5). Using this approach it was possible to trade stability and rise-time between the two channels (see Figure 8.4). This was not easily possible, however, for the Monte-Carlo runs where the design parameters were 'frozen'.

The SOFLC, in general, gave more active control signals, and in several cases approached limit cycle conditions. This is a well-known feature of fuzzy logic control. Although the scaling factors (three for each channel) had to be selected heuristically, this was greatly helped via previous experiments on engineering rigs. In particular, the switching regime of Figure 8.8, giving effectively coarse/fine control, produced a fast initial response together with good steady state accuracy. This regime also performed well on laboratory rigs. In nearly all the results, it can be seen that the SOFLC needed a second run to obtain a set of rules which would give good performance. This is not surprising, since the controller had an empty rule-base at the commencement of run 1 in each case. The second run also seemed necessary to obtain an adequate number of rules in the knowledge-base. Further runs beyond 3 seemed to extend the rule-base excessively and increase the computer burden. This has the implication that it would be desirable in a clinical setting to choose initial design values for the scaling factors and a tentative rule-base via prior simulation studies based on an average population model. Although the initial transient response was impressive, the steady state performance was inferior to that of GPC, as evidenced by the generally larger ITAE measures. A fast initial transient response is, however, an important issue in many operations since the surgeon wishes to commence procedures as soon as possible after patient entry into the operating theatre. In contrast, some deviation from set-point is tolerable particularly for the muscle relaxation channel.

It is difficult to make computational speed comparisons between the methods, since the studies were performed on different computing platforms. However, the SOFLC execution on a single T800 transputer was impressive. In fact, it was implemented in this way on a PC-hosted transputer system to enable multivariable SOFLC to be studied on a laboratory scale coupled electric drive rig, where a sampling period of 20 milliseconds was necessary (Linkens and Abbod, 1991). It performed adequately in this case.

The model utilised in this study was not truly multivariable, since it has only one-way interaction. It belongs to a category of systems known as triangular systems which does not necessarily render it easy to control. Although the structure of the model used considered the interactions in a feedforward manner by adopting a P-canonical form structure, other forms of control, such a feedforward compensation, could have been employed instead of feedback GPC and SOFLC. However, other drugs, especially inhalational anaesthetic agents, have different dynamic effects and hence the general feedback structure was retained for experimental comparisons. Also, other instances of multivariable control in biomedicine are being explored. One example is that of blood pressure management in intensive care, providing simultaneous control of blood pressure and cardiac output via simultaneous infusion of two drugs. Cases such as this give strongly cross-interactive systems for which GPC and SOFLC in full feedback configuration are necessary.

In conclusion it can be stated that self-adaptive strategies such as GPC give a superior control performance to a self-organising approach. It achieves this, however, from a detailed knowledge of the process dynamics. It has been assumed that the multivariable model used here is an accurate description of process structure, albeit with massive parameter uncertainty. In reality, such a model structure is at best an overdetermined abstraction, and therefore simplification, of life science systems. In the event of large structural uncertainties in process dynamics, the concept of self-organising control is attractive. This comparative study has shown it to be a tolerable runner-up in a situation which clearly favours the self-adaptive methodology. These conclusions are similar to those obtained by Al-Assaf (1988) who compared GPC and SOFLC applied to a cement grinding mill. He noted the need to apply a start-up signal to the process for obtaining suitable GPC paramount settings, and also the need for experimentation to fill the empty rule-base for SOFLC. His findings of inferior speed and steady state performance for SOFLC were based on single scaling factor settings. This contrast to the present study which used switched scaling factors to improve the performance via a 'course/fine' control strategy. Of course, we expect to see improvements in algorithms for both approaches. It is, however, in the area of self-organising control that we may expect to see more rapid advances in the future. The principle of SOFLC has been around for many years, but it still needs more detailed attention and comparison with its neural network equivalents which are currently fashionable. Recent work (Harris and Moore, 1990; Moore, 1991) has introduced the concept of Indirect SOFLC whereby a fuzzy model of the process is first identified, followed by inversion to provide a control algorithm. This is analogous to explicit self-tuning control, of which GPC is one example. It does, however, require *a priori* knowledge about the process in terms of its dynamical order, but provides self-organisation in terms of rules which allow for nonlinear situations.

CHAPTER NINE

Generalised Predictive Control with Pre-specified Set-points in Clinical Anaesthesia

9.1 Introduction

An advantage of predictive controllers in general and GPC in particular is the exploitation of the idea of pre-programmed or pre-specified set-points. Unlike other linear controllers, GPC allows for changes in the set-point profile, if known, to be communicated to the algorithm some samples ahead, thus giving the opportunity to the controller to adjust itself well before the changes take place. This interesting feature has proved very popular in areas of industry where the knowledge of these changes is possible. For instance, in robotics future arm trajectories can be known in advance, and in process industry, temperature profiles of furnaces for the treatment of special materials can also be known in advance. Similarly, during surgical operations in theatre the anaesthetist who is normally aware of the type of operation being performed, and therefore is also aware of the surgeon's future manipulations, can initiate changes in the patient's muscle relaxation level and depth of unconsciousness some time ahead of the surgeon's demands, leading therefore to a better interacting anaesthetic/surgical team. This is the theme of this chapter which is concerned with the application of the GPC algorithm together with pre-specified set-points in clinical anaesthesia. The study is divided into two parts; the first part deals with the application of the single-input single-output version of GPC to control muscle relaxation (paralysis) using two different patterns of set-points (with anticipated tolerances) for typical operations. These patterns were provided by an experienced anaesthetist (d'Hollander, 1992). The second part of the study concerns the extension of the above work to the multivariable case involving simultaneous control of muscle relaxation together with unconsciousness through blood pressure measurements (see Chapter 4).

9.2 SISO GPC and the set-point pre-specification concept

Let us recall the result of the minimisation of the cost function described by equation (2.12) as given by equation (2.20):

$$\Delta u(t) = \bar{g}^T(\omega - \Psi)$$

where $\Psi = [\Psi(t + N_1), \ldots, \Psi(t + N_2)]$, $\bar{g}^T$ is the first row of the matrix $(G_d^T G_d + \lambda I)^{-1} G_d^T$, and G_d is the dynamic (step-response) matrix of the form given in Clarke *et al.* (1987a).

In order to introduce the pre-specified or pre-programmed set-points into the calculations of GPC, the future set-point trajectory ω is used to calculate the future set-point errors. This feature, which is not available in other single stage algorithms such as GMV, consists of minimising the difference between the range of future predictions and trajectory of future set-points $\omega(t) = [\omega_1, \omega_2, \ldots, \omega_{N2}]^T$ instead of a constant set-point $\omega(t) = \omega$ for $t = 1, 2, \ldots, N_2$. Thus, at time t the control calculation procedure may be forced to take into account set-point changes occurring N_2 samples in the future. For instance, if a set-point change is likely to occur, say, at sample time 100 then the controller output starts reacting to this change at sample time $100 - N_2$. As already mentioned, such a feature is widely available in process control and robot control applications where better performances have been reported, but the most important benefits can be experienced in multivariable applications where improved decoupling is expected, as will be shown in later sections. It is, however, worth mentioning that when the prediction horizon has to be chosen large, in either SISO or MIMO systems, smoother control actions are to be expected and if tighter control is required, the control horizon NU should be chosen larger than 1; this is due to the fact that the controller needs more degrees of freedom to choose the appropriate control sequence. In fact, it can be shown that for large N_2 and large NU the GPC solution tends to the simpler LQ controller and a general guideline suggests that for a sampling time of 0.2 to 0.1 the settling-time of the plant, the knowledge of 10 future samples is usually adequate to obtain a good response.

9.3 Simulation results

The simulation study considered the continuous model described by equations (2.8) and (2.7) with the exception that the open-loop gain was increased to 2.5. A fourth-order Runge–Kutta method was used with a fixed step length of 0.1 and a sampling interval of 1 minute. An initial high level of 15 (units) was applied for one sample in order to mimic the initial bolus injection normally administered by anaesthetists in theatre. During that period the loop was open and remained so until the output (paralysis level) reached the safety level of 90% when the loop was closed with a fixed PI whose parameters had been selected for an average patient population. This form of control was operational until sample time 25 min when the adaptive GPC took over with the following parameters:

$$N_1 = 1, \quad N_2 = 10, \quad NU = 1, \quad \lambda = 1.0$$

$$P(z^{-1}) = 1.0, \quad T(z^{-1}) = (1 - 0.8z^{-1})^2$$

The set-points changes were known to the algorithm N_2 samples in advance.

For parameter estimation a UD-factorisation method was used with an initial covariance matrix of $Cov = 10^3 . I$ and a forgetting factor of $\rho = 0.95$. A third-order model of 3 a's and 3 b's with an assumed time delay of 1 minute was estimated starting at sample time 20 minutes (the time at which the nonlinear region has already been traversed) with the following initial values:

$\hat{a}_1 = -2.419$

$\hat{a}_2 = 1.939$

$\hat{a}_3 = -0.516$

$\hat{b}_1 = 1.07 \ 10^{-02}$

$\hat{b}_2 = -1.44 \ 10^{-03}$

$\hat{b}_3 = -6.81 \ 10^{-03}$

The data measurement vector included positional data as well as filtered incremental data. The experiments conducted were based on two different patterns of set-points which correspond to classical abdominal surgery procedures such as cholecystectomy by laparoscopy, and a gastroplasty for hiatus hernia, which are relatively common.

- *Pattern A: for cholecystectomy*

    1. Step 1 As fast as possible (5 min) to an EMG of 15%.
    2. Step 2 Maintaining EMG level at 15% for 60 min $\pm$ 20 min.
    3. Step 3 Moving to an EMG level of 40 $\pm$ 5% within 10 $\pm$ 2 min.
    4. Step 4 Maintaining the EMG level at 40 $\pm$ 5% for 10 min.

- *Pattern B: for gastroplasty*

    1. Step 1 As fast as possible (5 min) to an EMG of 15%.
    2. Step 2 Maintaining EMG level at 15% for 150 min $\pm$ 30 min.
    3. Step 3 Moving to an EMG level of 25 $\pm$ 5% within 10 $\pm$ 2 min.
    4. Step 4 Maintaining the EMG level at 25 $\pm$ 5% for 60 min $\pm$ 10 min.
    5. Step 5 Moving to an EMG level of 40 $\pm$ 5% within 10 $\pm$ 2 min.
    6. Step 6 Maintaining the EMG level of 40 $\pm$ 5% for 30 min.

The simulations were undertaken in two parts; the first part considered using the matched case between the pre-programmed set-point and the actual one, whereas the second part considered the mismatch case between the two.

9.3.1 Experiments in the matched case

The first experiment involved using the algorithm on the model with nominal values (no tolerances) for the set-points of '*Pattern A*'. Using filtered incremental data for the measurement vector in the estimator led to the result shown in Figure 9.1 where

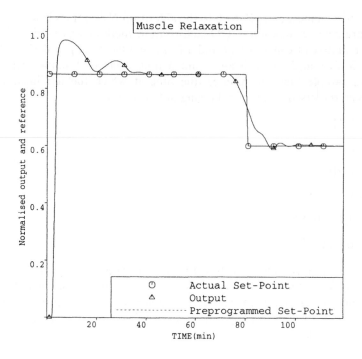

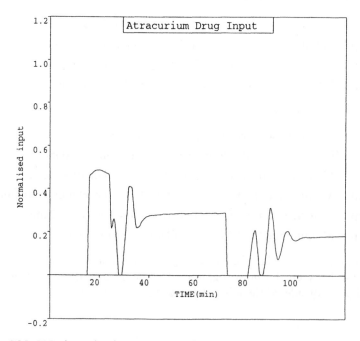

Figure 9.1   SISO GPC of muscle relaxation for a typical set-point profile corresponding to a cholecystectomy (*Pattern A*) surgical operation; incremental data-type for estimation. Matched case.

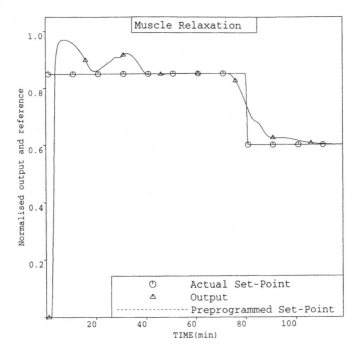

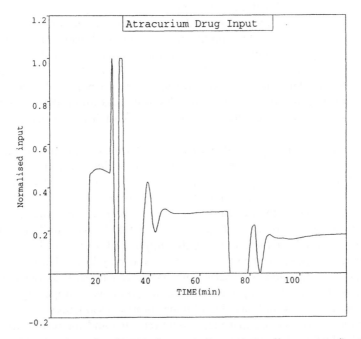

Figure 9.2   SISO GPC of muscle relaxation for a typical set-point profile corresponding to a cholecystectomy (*Pattern A*) surgical operation; positional data-type for estimation. Matched case.

it can be seen that the output tracked the set-point adequately without any under-shoot (which is undesirable in operating theatres) with a reasonable control activity. The output did not reach the initial set-point within the 5 minutes specified but the fact that no undershoot was produced suggests the overall performance can be considered as acceptable. When positional data were fed to the estimator rather than incremental, the performance of Figure 9.2 shows that the control signal saturated when GPC took over from the fixed PI controller leading therefore to a significant overshoot during the first set-point phase, suggesting that data filtering is essential. Also, due to this large initial overshoot, the time to reach an EMG of 15% (output of 0.85) was significantly larger than in the previous case.

When '*pattern B*' was considered, using incremental data led to the performance of Figure 9.3 where, despite the set-point changes occurring at short time intervals, the controller behaved well again with reasonable control activity. The use of positional data for the measurement vector in the estimator led to the performance of Figure 9.4 where it can be seen that except for the saturation of the input signal during the initial set-point phase, the performance was comparable with that of Figure 9.3.

9.3.2   Experiments in the mismatch case

As has been mentioned before, the experienced anaesthetist can anticipate the surgeon's manipulations and accommodate for them by forcing the controller to react well in advance of those set-point profile changes. However, it is possible that the surgeon changes his mind and/or introduces a new element during surgery which can override those anticipated set-point profiles. This is the theme of this section which considers the same scenario using the set-point tolerances and time constraints given above. It is worth noting that only maximum tolerances have been considered in this study since the reader is able to visualise what happens in other cases.

The first experiment considered '*Pattern A*' but with a set-point profile given by the maximum tolerances as shown in Figure 9.5 in which the controller was given the nominal tolerances, whereas the actual set-point changes occurred later. Using filtered incremental data for the estimator the experiment led to the performance of Figure 9.6 where, due to the early reaction of the controller, the output managed to converge to the new set-point at the time of set-point change. Similarly, when positional data were used for the estimator, the output of Figure 9.7 also behaved well by tracking the set-point at the set-point changes. It may be argued that in this case the output's early reaction to a set-point change can be seen as detrimental, but because in both cases the approach to the set-point was happening in a rather smooth fashion, it would not have led to undesirable consequences.

For '*Pattern B*', the same experiments were repeated and the results are shown in Figures 9.8 and 9.9 for incremental data and positional data respectively.

Finally, Table 9.1 summarises the time performances of the algorithm in reaching the set-points for patterns A and B and it can be seen that except for the initial set-point, the subsequent time constraints are achievable without too much compromise on other constraints such as output tolerances and control signal activity.

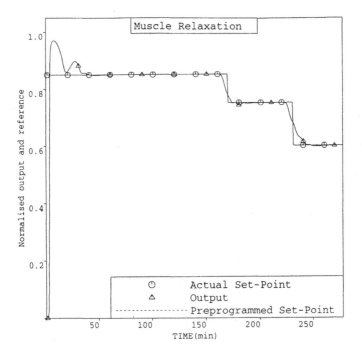

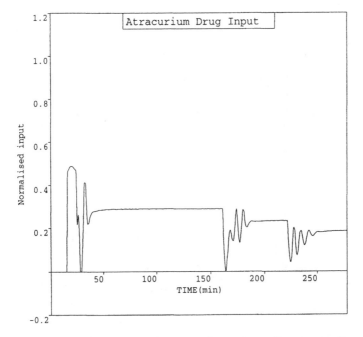

Figure 9.3 SISO GPC of muscle relaxation for a typical set-point profile corresponding to a gastroplasty (*Pattern B*) surgical operation; incremental data-type for estimation. Matched case.

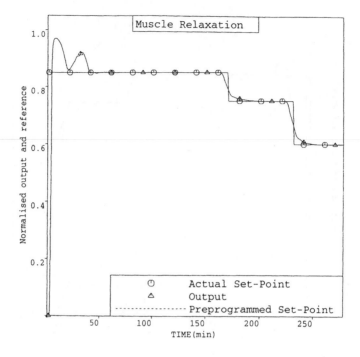

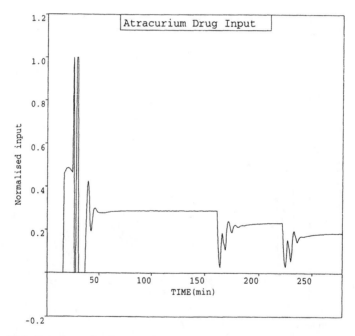

Figure 9.4   SISO GPC of muscle relaxation for a typical set-point profile corresponding to a gastroplasty (*Pattern B*) surgical operation; positional data-type for estimation. Matched case.

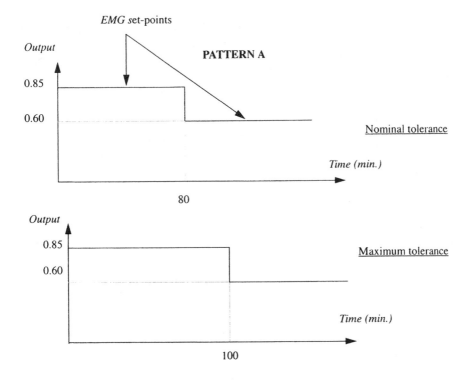

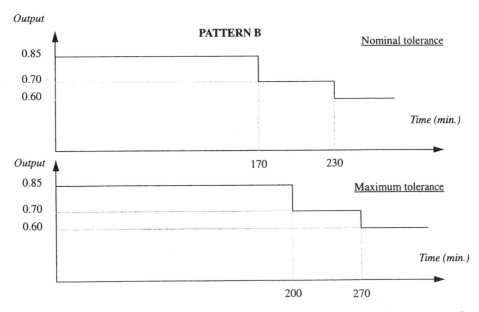

Figure 9.5 Diagrammatic representation of the various set-point tolerances within *Pattern A* and *Pattern B* set-point profiles.

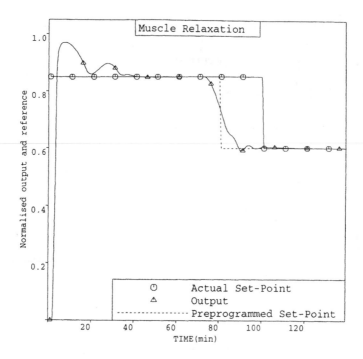

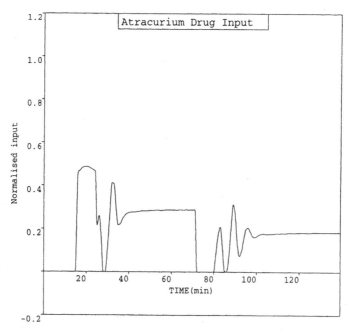

Figure 9.6 SISO GPC of muscle relaxation for a typical set-point profile corresponding to a cholecystectomy (*Pattern A*) surgical operation; incremental data-type for estimation. Set-point mismatch case.

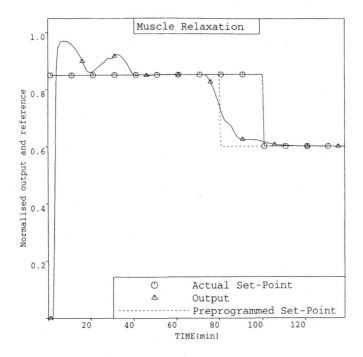

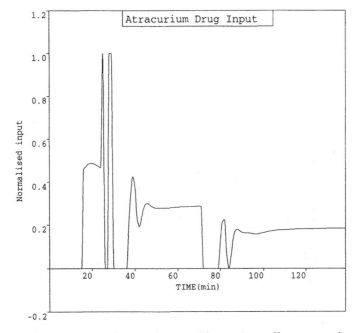

Figure 9.7 SISO GPC of muscle relaxation for a typical set-point profile corresponding to a cholecystectomy (*Pattern A*) surgical operation; positional data-type for estimation. Set-point mismatch case.

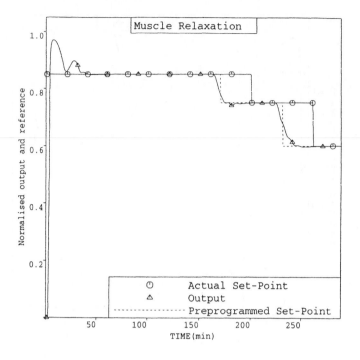

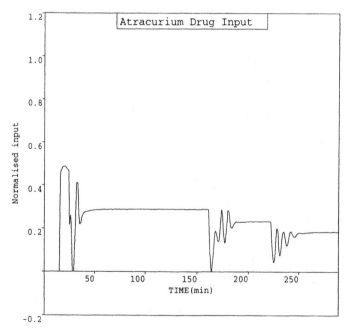

Figure 9.8   SISO GPC of muscle relaxation for a typical set-point profile corresponding to a gastroplasty (*Pattern B*) surgical operation; incremental data-type for estimation. Set-point mismatch case.

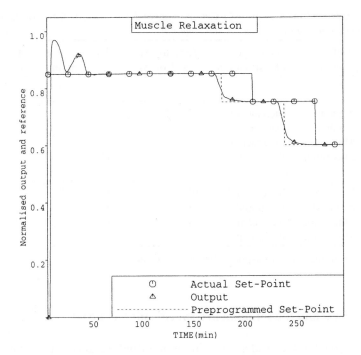

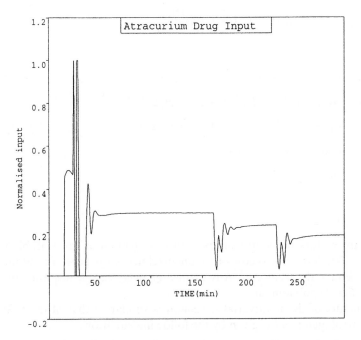

Figure 9.9 SISO GPC of muscle relaxation for a typical set-point profile corresponding to a gastroplasty (*Pattern B*) surgical operation; positional data-type for estimation. Set-point mismatch case.

Table 9.1 Time performances of SISO GPC in satisfying the anaesthetist's constraints for the set-point profiles referred to as *Pattern A* and *Pattern B*

Figure number	Profile tolerance	Data-type for estimation	Time to reach step 1 (min)	Time to reach step 2 (min)	Time to reach step 3 (min)
Pattern A					
9.1	Nominal	Incremental	19	8	–
9.2	Nominal	Positional	25	23	–
9.6	Maximum	Incremental	19	1*	–
9.7	Maximum	Positional	25	1*	–
Pattern B					
9.3	Nominal	Incremental	19	2	10
9.4	Nominal	Positional	25	8	9
9.8	Maximum	Incremental	19	1*	1*
9.9	Maximum	Positional	25	1*	1*

* Evaluated from the time of set-point change occurrence.

9.4 MIMO GPC and the set-point pre-specification concept

Similarly to Chapter 4, consider the m-input m-output linear discrete-time system:

$$A(z^{-1})Y(t) = B(z^{-1})U(t-1) + \frac{C(z^{-1})\xi(t)}{\Delta} \qquad (9.1)$$

where

$$A(z^{-1}) = I + A_1 z^{-1} + A_2 z^{-2} + \ldots + A_n z^{-n}$$

$$B(z^{-1}) = B_1 + B_2 z^{-1} + B_3 z^{-2} + \ldots + B_s z^{-s+1}$$

$$C(z^{-1}) = C_0 + C_1 z^{-1} + C_2 z^{-2} + \ldots + C_p z^{-p}$$

$$Y(t) = [y_1(t), y_2(t), \ldots, y_m(t)]$$

$$U(t) = [u_1(t), u_2(t), \ldots, u_m(t)]$$

and

$$\Delta = 1 - z^{-1}$$

$Y(t)$, $U(t)$ are vectors of 'm' measurable outputs $y(t)$ and 'm' measurable inputs $u(t)$ respectively. $\xi(t)$ denotes a vector of 'm' uncorrelated sequences of random variables with zero mean and variance σ^2. Any extra time delay can be absorbed in the structure of the $B(z^{-1})$ polynomial.

The structure of the multivariable version is similar to that of the SISO version and the control increment is given by the following equation:

$$\Delta U(t) = \bar{G}^T(\omega - \Psi) \qquad (9.2)$$

It is common knowledge that when dealing with multivariable structures the problem of decoupling between the various loops is crucial. Early work by other researchers (Kam *et al.*, 1985) focused on the idea of representing the loops cross-coupling in a feedforward manner by considering the so-called P-canonical form for

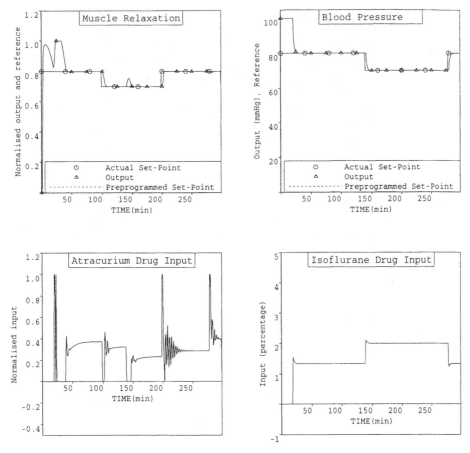

Figure 9.10 Multivariable GPC for anaesthesia without set-point pre-specification; $N_1 = 1$, $N_2 = 10$, NU(ch 1) $= 2$, NU(ch 2) $= 1$, $P(z^{-1}) = T(z^{-1}) = I$.

equation (9.1), implying that the process outputs are only affected by the various inputs. In fact, several studies showed that such a model representation, indeed, improves decoupling considerably. In the case of GPC, there has been much published work in relation to decoupling properties (Mohtadi, 1986; Mohtadi *et al.*, 1992). It emerged from this work and others that low and medium frequency decoupling can be reduced by using the model-following polynomial $P(z^{-1})$ which enables the reduction of the closed-loop frequency bandwidth. Most effectively, however, decoupling can be achieved by introducing the set-points in advance enabling therefore the system to be fully decoupled although it is widely agreed that some form of interaction is sometimes needed.

The simulation studies considered the continuous anaesthetic model described in Chapter 4. A fourth-order Runge–Kutta method was used with a fixed step length of 0.1 and a sampling interval of 1 minute. For parameter estimation a UD-factorisation method was used on incremental data with initial covariance matrix and forgetting factor given by: $P = 10^2 . I$ and $\rho = 0.975$, respectively. A multivariable model of 5 diagonal $A(z^{-1})$ matrices together with 5 upper triangular

$B(z^{-1})$ matrices was estimated (see Chapter 4) with an assumed time delay of 1 minute. Initial conditions were 0% relaxation and 100 mmHg arterial pressure. The set-point command signal was 80% then 70% for relaxation, and 80 mmHg then 70 mmHg for the blood pressure. Set-point changes in both channels were known to the algorithm N_2 samples ahead. A bolus dose of atracurium of 67 mg at 1 mg ml^{-1} concentration was initially applied for one sample while the isoflurane input was kept at 0. While the bolus effect took place, the loop remained open until the output in the muscle relaxation channel reached the safety level of 85%, when the loop was closed. The self-tuner was allowed to run with the initial parameter estimates until sample time 39 min when the parameter estimation routine was allowed to be operational. The adopted GPC tuning knobs were as follows: $N_1 = 1$; $N_2 = 10$; NU (ch 1) = 2; NU (ch 2) = 1; $P = T = I$, where I is the matrix identity.

The first experiment considered the multivariable GPC without set-point pre-specification. The result of the run is shown in Figure 9.10 where the output response of channel 1 (i.e. paralysis) demonstrated some interaction at sample time 140 min where there was a set-point change in the unconsciousness channel.

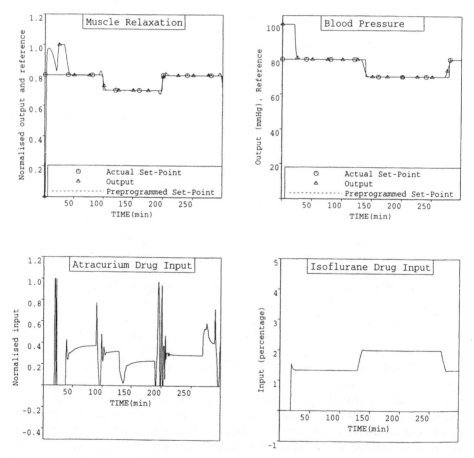

Figure 9.11   Multivariable GPC for anaesthesia with set-point pre-specification; $N_1 = 1$, $N_2 = 10$, NU(ch 1) = 2, NU(ch 2) = 1, $P(z^{-1}) = T(z^{-1}) = I$.

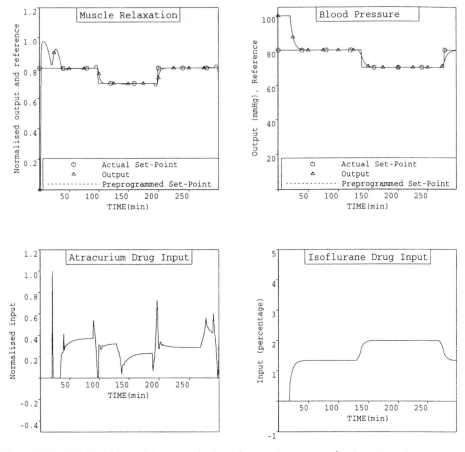

Figure 9.12 Multivariable GPC for anaesthesia with set-point pre-specification; $N_1 = 1$, $N_2 = 10$, NU(ch 1) = 2, NU(ch 2) = 1,

$$P(z^{-1}) = \begin{bmatrix} \dfrac{(1 - 0.7z^{-1})}{0.3} & 0 \\ & \dfrac{(1 - 0.9z^{-1})}{0.1} \\ 0 & \end{bmatrix}, \quad T(z^{-1}) = (1 - 0.8z^{-1})^2 . I.$$

However, when the set-point changes were specified to the algorithm in advance the system was fully decoupled as seen in Figure 9.11. Also, the use of

$$P(z^{-1}) = \begin{bmatrix} \dfrac{(1 - 0.7z^{-1})}{0.3} & 0 \\ & (1 - 0.9z^{-1}) \\ 0 & \dfrac{}{0.1} \end{bmatrix}$$

and $T(z^{-1}) = (1 - 0.8z^{-1})^2 . I$ for control and estimation in the experiment of Figure 9.12 shows how the system can stay decoupled while the response speed can be tailored to one's specifications, for instance slowing it down in the second channel and keeping it fast in the first. Finally, the last experiment considered a mismatch between the programmed set-point and the actual set-point in channel 1. As shown in Figure 9.13 the performance is acceptable since the output tracked the set-point

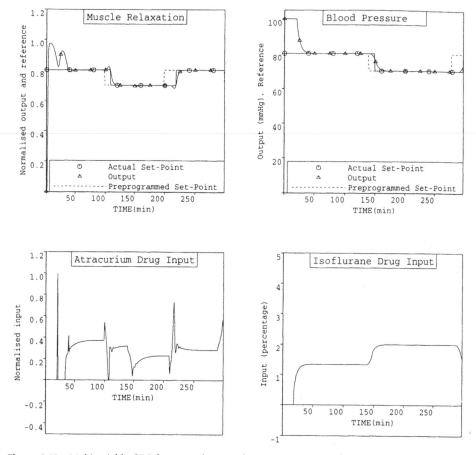

Figure 9.13 Multivariable GPC for anaesthesia with set-point pre-specification; $N_1 = 1$, $N_2 = 10$, $NU(\text{ch 1}) = 2$, $NU(\text{ch 2}) = 1$,

$$P(z^{-1}) = \begin{bmatrix} (1 - 0.7z^{-1}) & 0 \\ 0.3 & (1 - 0.9z^{-1}) \\ 0 & 0.1 \end{bmatrix}, \quad T(z^{-1}) = (1 - 0.8z^{-1})^2 . I. \text{ Set-point mismatch case.}$$

without too much delay, although the controller reacted too early to the set-point changes.

9.5   Conclusions

In light of the experiments described in this chapter, it can be said that the use of pre-specified set-points, be it in single-loop or multi-loop systems, can considerably contribute to improving the closed-loop characteristics of such systems. In the study, it has been established that:

1.   If the set-point profile for muscle relaxation is known within certain tolerances, the algorithm can lead to good results even if mismatches between the actual and the programmed profiles exist.

2. As already emphasised in Chapter 2, during clinical trials either positional data or incremental data can be used for the measurement (information) vector in the estimator for updating the patient model with good performances as a result (profile constraints achievable).

3. When the system is extended to the multivariable case involving simultaneous control of muscle relaxation and unconsciousness by means of blood pressure measurements, full decoupling can be realised without affecting too much the system's ability to fulfil other important objectives such as good tracking abilities, reasonable control activity, etc.

Supervisory Generalised Predictive Control and Fault Detection for Multivariable Anaesthesia

10.1 Introduction

In the field of biomedicine, the theme of self-tuning controllers is very advantageous because of the large patient-to-patient variations in kinetics parameters. In fact, early work conducted by pioneers in this research field (Sheppard *et al.*, 1979; Linkens *et al.*, 1981; Zhang and Cameron, 1989) demonstrated through clinical experiments on humans that this form of control is effective and most importantly safe. While the superiority of this form of control is directly linked to the complexity of the associated control algorithm, the overall strategy which includes initial tuning and self-adaptation cannot pretend to the name of *autonomous* control unless diagnosis and supervision are added to current existing features (autonomous controllers implying here self-governing controllers) (Astrom, 1992). Such an ambitious scheme would not be possible without the availability of increasing computational capabilities. Because of the existence of this latter capability, there is growing demand for **fault tolerance** which is not only achievable through improvements to the components included in the corresponding control system, but also by using a hierarchical supervisory level for fault tolerance management. This would detect a fault early enough to avoid later emerging signs of complications, isolate it and accommodate it, all of this by using a so-called fault detection isolation accommodation (FDIA) scheme. This latter scheme is considered nowadays to form an integral part of an automatic control system in situations where a variety of faults can be expected. Moreover, while the surgeons are performing their manipulations in operating theatres, safety is usually given top priority via continuous monitoring of different variables such as blood pressure, heart rate, respiration rate, etc., together with the checks that are frequently done on the equipment connected to the patient. Alarms are usually fitted to all apparatus, and are triggered only when a particular variable goes out of bounds. This is particularly the theme of this research study which considers an analytical redundancy algorithm for the detection, isolation and accommodation of faults that are to be expected in intensive care units and particularly during simultaneous control of muscle relaxation via atracurium intravenous injection and unconsciousness via isoflurane inhalation (see Chapter 4). Hence, the redundancy algorithm is coupled with multivariable GPC using a P-canonical form (see Chapter 4) or multivariable GPC with feedforward (multivariable GPCF) (see Chapter 6) to form an integrated system which will be able to fulfil control, adaptation and monitoring simultaneously on the multivariable anaesthesia control system reviewed previously. The study is organised into the following sections: Section 10.2 reviews the various faults associated with the control system. Section 10.3 summarises the structure of the algorithm associated with the hierarchical layer, whereas Section 10.4 describes the simulation experiments. Finally, constructive conclusions from this study are drawn in Section 10.5 together with an outline of future work.

10.2   A review of faults associated with the multivariable control system

With reference to Figure 4.2 representing the multivariable anaesthesia control system, the faults associated with the system can be divided into two blocks: the first block relates to the atracurium/muscle relaxation path, whereas the second concerns the isoflurane/mean arterial pressure path. However, various failures in each block can be of three types sensor failures, actuator failures and algorithmic failures. The following sections describe each of them in more detail.

10.2.1   Sensor failures

These are mainly due to the Relaxograph device which is responsible for EMG recordings and the Dinamap instrument which provides blood pressure measurements. Diathermy (which produces an electrical interference) as well as movements of the patient's arm during surgery can also cause false readings as follows.

Diathermy

This causes the EMG level to drop by more than 5% of its current value for one sample or more.

Movement of the patient's arm during surgery

In the muscle relaxation channel the patient's arm movement causes a sudden shift in the EMG level of more than 5% of its current value for more than two samples if the movement is permanent, and less if it is a recoverable one. In the blood pressure channel this movement induces a shift in the arterial pressure of more than 5 mmHg.

10.2.2   Actuator failures

The actuator, being typified in this case by a syringe pump unit and responsible for administering atracurium through an infusion line, can sometimes fail to fulfil this task due to a breakdown or to a communication error. The result is a slow and continuous rise in the recorded EMG to an unacceptable level.

10.2.3   Algorithmic failures

Another type of failure that can occur in such circumstances is a failure in the actual algorithm responsible for the control strategy, in this case the self-adaptive GPC. As the word 'adaptive' implies, two interdependent tasks are involved; a recursive parameter estimation and a control law calculation.

A fault in the estimator

Although faults associated with a recursive parameter estimator scheme can be numerous those associated with covariance matrix are the most usual ones. Indeed, in cases where limits are imposed on the control signals, as soon as the adaptation starts, unreasonable controller outputs are generated. A check on the covariance trace ($\sum P_{jj}$) would prove that the estimator has incorrectly learned the process.

A fault in the control law

As a result of the previous estimator failure or a wrong choice of the GPC tuning knobs, the closed-loop poles can be badly located in the z-plane leading therefore to unstable or oscillatory modes.

10.3   The hierarchical supervisory level: structure and algorithm

The overall multivariable anaesthesia control system represented in Figure 4.2 has been given an intelligent or autonomous structure by superimposing on top of the multivariable GPC level a supervisory layer that will have the task of monitoring and assessing its performance at every sample as Figure 10.1 illustrates. To be chronologically related, the sequence of events within this layer would be as follows.

Just after the initial bolus injection, initial parameter estimates which will normally enable the GPC algorithm to run during its initial stages are chosen on the basis of two procedures in the gain scheduling block; the first of these procedures estimates the patient's gain to atracurium, while the second estimates this patient's gain to isoflurane. The control algorithm is then allowed to run assuming these parameter values for a few samples. At the same time the signals' validity block starts to operate by ensuring that both the EMG and the mean arterial pressure (MAP) signals are within certain pre-specified ranges. When it is judged that reasonable data have been gathered from the loop, the parameter estimation routine is triggered. Once a normal state of operation is reached, the FDIA algorithm is made operational. If a fault is detected according to a certain criterion, checks on the absolute signals and their trends are run to isolate the fault and issue appropriate display and audible warnings and alarms, and at the same time, depending on the fault type, a decision is taken upon which compensatory measures to adopt in such circumstances. Also, while the adaptation is on, a check on the integrity of the

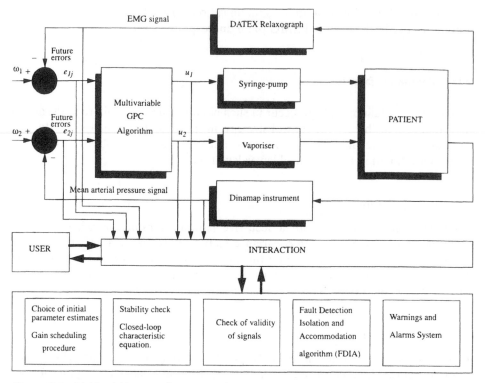

Figure 10.1   Multivariable anaesthesia control system including hierarchical supervisory level.

parameter estimator is run together with an analysis of the closed-loop character-istic equation. The following sections review briefly the different main blocks in more detail.

10.3.1   The gain scheduling block

Estimation of the patient's gain to atracurium

Neglecting the time delay let us rewrite the linear part of the mathematical model associated with the drug atracurium (equation (2.8)):

$$G_{11}(s) = \frac{K_{atr}(1 + T_4 s)}{(1 + T_1 s)(1 + T_2 s)(1 + T_3 s)}$$

or

$$\begin{cases} G_{11}(s) = \dfrac{K_{atr} T_4}{T_1 T_2 T_3} \left[\dfrac{s + a}{(s + b)(s + c)(s + d)} \right] \\[2mm] a = \dfrac{1}{T_4}; \ b = \dfrac{1}{T_1}; \ c = \dfrac{1}{T_2}; \ d = \dfrac{1}{T_3} \end{cases} \tag{10.1}$$

Considering that the bolus dose is equivalent to an impulse response and including the Hill equation (2.7) and taking the inverse Laplace transform, it follows that:

$$K_{atr} = \left[\frac{y}{1-y}\right]^{1/\alpha} D \frac{T_1 T_2 T_3}{T_4 u(t)[A\ e^{-bt} + B\ e^{-ct} + C\ e^{-dt}]} \qquad (10.2)$$

where A, B and C are constants depending on the quantities a, b, c and d and given by the following expressions:

$$A = (s+b)G_{11}(s)\Big|_{s=-b} = \frac{(a-b)}{(c-b)(d-b)}$$

$$B = (s+c)G_{11}(s)\Big|_{s=-c} = \frac{(a-c)}{(b-c)(d-c)}$$

$$C = (s+d)G_{11}(s)\Big|_{s=-d} = \frac{(a-d)}{(b-d)(c-d)}$$

Using the following nominal values for the various variables:

$$\begin{cases} T_1 = 3.08 \text{ min} \\ T_2 = 4.81 \text{ min} \\ T_3 = 34.42 \text{ min} \\ T_4 = 10.64 \text{ min} \\ \alpha = 2.98 \\ D = 0.404 \end{cases}$$

it follows that:

$$K_{atr} = \left[\frac{y}{1-y}\right]^{1/2.98} \left[\frac{19.36}{-6.68\ e^{-0.32t} + 5.45\ e^{-0.21t} + 1.23\ e^{-0.03t}}\right]\frac{1}{u(t)} \qquad (10.3)$$

The values y and t can be obtained from the transient response at the peak values. Three intervals were chosen to assign regions for the parameter estimates:

$$0.5 \leq K_{atr\ low} < 1.5$$

$$1.5 \leq K_{atr\ medium} < 2.5 \qquad (10.4)$$

$$2.5 \leq K_{atr\ high} < 3.5$$

Estimation of the patient's gain to isoflurane

In earlier published work (Millard *et al.*, 1988a, 1988b), it has been reported that step response trials using isoflurane were performed on patients 20 minutes before surgery commenced in order to determine how sensitive these patients were to the drug; this is common practice in theatres before surgery commences. Knowing that the responses obey first-order characteristics, i.e. if a 1% step input of isoflurane is applied then it follows that:

$$K_{iso} = [MAP_f - MAP_i] \qquad (10.5)$$

Here also it has been decided to use three categories for the patient's gain to iso-flurane:

$$-20 \leq K_{\text{iso low}} < -14$$
$$-14 \leq K_{\text{iso medium}} < -12 \tag{10.6}$$
$$-12 \leq K_{\text{iso high}} < -10$$

10.3.2 Signals' validity block

EMG and MAP signals are checked against three regions; safe, caution and alarm as Figure 10.2 shows. Hence, three flags were used to define a particular status, i.e.:

Safe = Green flag

Caution = Orange flag

Alarm = Red flag

The flags can be given binary numbers. Table 10.1 shows the nine possible combinations that could be obtained.

10.3.3 Estimator's integrity block

In order to protect the estimation from learning the process too well and consequently converging to values that do not verify the certainty equivalence principle, a check on the traces of the covariance matrices in both channels ensures that these values do not fall below a certain acceptable threshold.

10.3.4 Fault detection isolation accommodation (FDIA) block

The general structure of a process fault detection method is represented in Figure 10.3 (Isermann, 1984). It makes use of non-measurable quantities and therefore is based on a process model. The control strategy based on the GPC algorithm uses a model of the process explicitly to calculate the parameters of its corresponding control law.

Table 10.1 Decision table for signals' validity flags

Status number	Flags' status						Region
	$Flgr_1$	$Flgr_2$	$Flor_1$	$Flor_2$	$Flrd_1$	$Flrd_2$	
1	1	1	0	0	0	0	Safe
2	1	0	0	1	0	0	Caution
3	1	0	0	0	0	1	Alarm
4	0	1	1	0	0	0	Caution
5	0	1	0	0	1	0	Alarm
6	0	0	1	1	0	0	Caution
7	0	0	0	0	1	1	Alarm
8	0	0	1	0	0	1	Alarm
9	0	0	0	1	1	0	Alarm

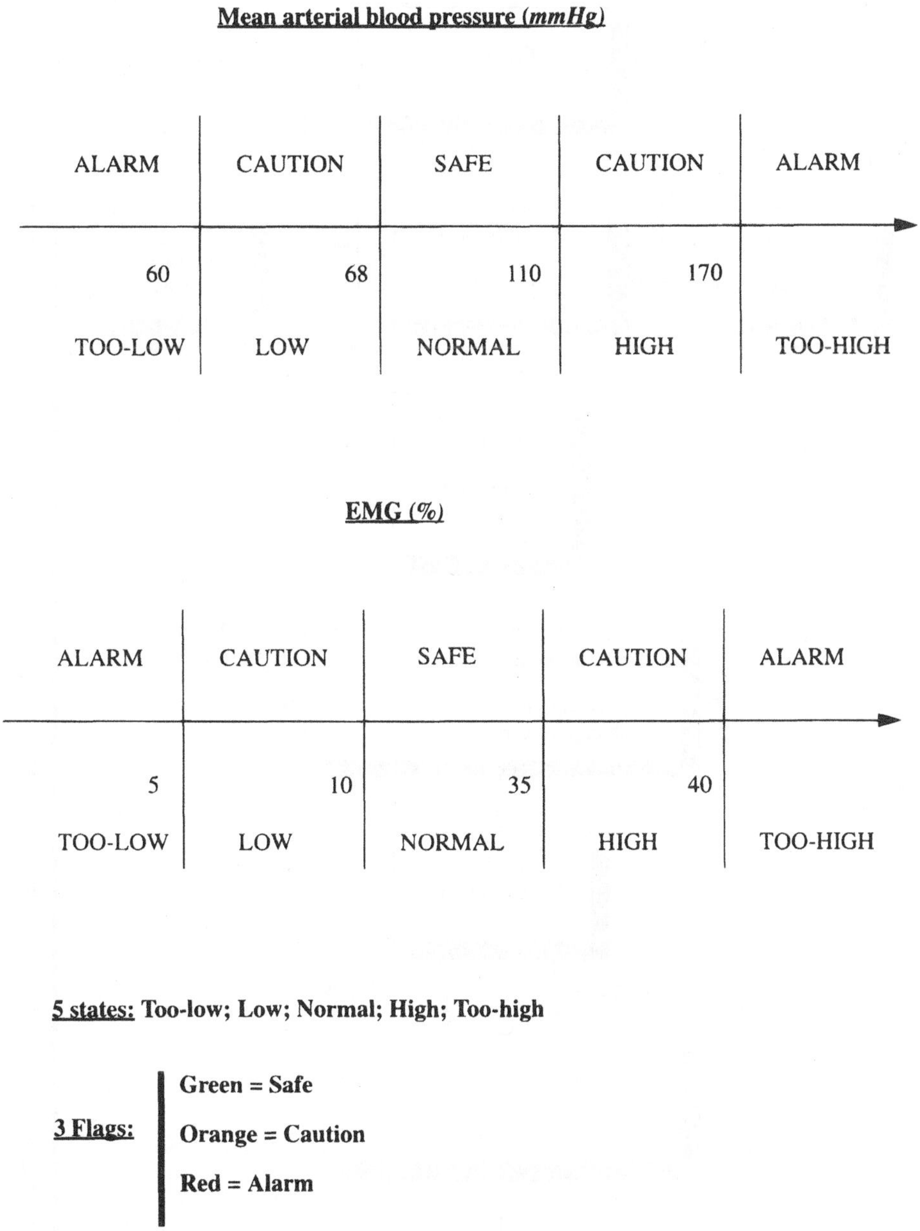

Mean arterial blood pressure (*mmHg*)

ALARM	CAUTION	SAFE	CAUTION	ALARM
60	68	110	170	
TOO-LOW	LOW	NORMAL	HIGH	TOO-HIGH

EMG (%)

ALARM	CAUTION	SAFE	CAUTION	ALARM
5	10	35	40	
TOO-LOW	LOW	NORMAL	HIGH	TOO-HIGH

5 states: Too-low; Low; Normal; High; Too-high

3 Flags:
Green = Safe
Orange = Caution
Red = Alarm

Figure 10.2 Definition of signal validity zones for blood pressure and EMG signals.

Briefly summarised, the FDIA algorithm consists of three models: a model of the **normal** process, a model of the **observed** process, and a model of the **faulty** process. The normal state is widely defined as the state which just precedes an alarmed fault, implying that the user must be aware of the 'normal' allowable tolerances (Isermann, 1984). The models of the faulty process show the effects of the faults on the chosen analysed quantities, the effects being called 'fault signatures'.

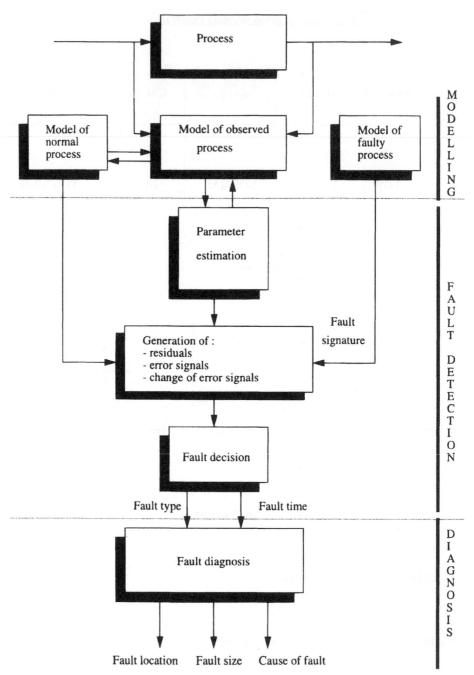

Figure 10.3   Structure of an FDI method based on non-measurable quantities.

Detection

Since the structure of GPC inherently possesses an identification mechanism, it is beneficial to adopt the process model-based method for detection. The model-based method uses the least number of sensors to monitor the operating state of the system (Isermann, 1984). Being based on a linearised discrete-time model any non-linearity is linearised.

Consider a healthy model and its prediction error (residual):

$$A(z^{-1})\tilde{y}(t) = B(z^{-1})u(t) + x(t) \tag{10.7}$$

and

$$|\tilde{\varepsilon}| = |\tilde{y} - \hat{\theta}\Phi^T| \tag{10.8}$$

where $\tilde{y}$ is the observed output, $\hat{\theta}$ the estimates, Φ the measurement vector which includes the input–output information.

For a healthy system, there is no estimated model mismatch, leading therefore to an almost zero residual. Any non-zero residual comes from persistently exciting noise, components aging, etc. The effect of these uncertainties causes the residual to deviate from the zero baseline, however, it is limited within some pre-defined threshold.

Now consider a faulty model and its residual as follows:

$$[A(z^{-1}) + \Delta A(z^{-1})]\tilde{y}(t) = [B(z^{-1}) + \Delta B(z^{-1})]u(t) \tag{10.9}$$

and

$$|\tilde{\varepsilon}| = \tilde{y} + \Delta y - \Phi^T(\hat{\theta} + \Delta\hat{\theta}) \tag{10.10}$$

where ΔA and ΔB represent the discrepancies due to the changes in the system structures, Δy may be due to failure caused by bias of the sensors or disturbances acting on the system, and $\Delta\hat{\theta}$ denotes a fault in the system structure and faults in the state variable sensors. Hence, when a fault occurs, the value of $|\tilde{\varepsilon}|$ in equation (10.10) will be greater than that of equation (10.8); this forms the basis for the fault detection mechanism used throughout, i.e. the residual value is checked against a preset threshold drawn from the **normal** state of operation. The main difficulty which lies with this methodology is the selection of the threshold value. Choosing it too low would increase the rate of false alarms, and conversely setting it too high would increase the rate of fault misses. Therefore a compromise has to be made in choosing this value. At this stage it is worth noting that the use of a separate estimator for each loop will allow one to treat the loops separately by calculating and testing their corresponding residuals.

Isolation (diagnosis)

In order to isolate (diagnose) a fault, Isermann (1984) converted the estimated parameters into system coefficients. In this study we found it difficult to make an inference using this conversion method. Instead, we used another way of isolating a fault by running checks on the absolute signals and their trends (Isermann, 1981). For the absolute signals, a check is made on the evolution of the error signal *Reference – Output* over a window length of k samples. Here again threshold values have to be supplied which set tolerance bands. Two signal categories can be defined: low and high, and a check on the absolute signal trend *Present output – Past output*

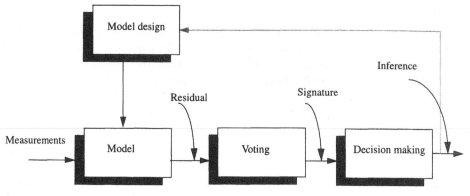

Figure 10.4   Stages of model-based fault detection and diagnosis.

would confirm or deny the existence of a particular fault. Here also, thresholds have to be specified by the user for the two signal categories which again can be defined as low and high. It is worth noting that the detected variables can result from a combination of faults and noise. Because the assumption of a purely deterministic system is not a realistic one, it is necessary to separate noise from the testing signals by adopting the idea of voting, as shown in Figure 10.4, in which the particular fault occurs m samples out of k samples in the *a priori* chosen window ($m < k$).

Flags are provided for $|Error|$, $|Error\ rate|$ and trace and are set to 0 or 1 depending on whether a certain proposition is false or true. For instance, if the absolute value of error is greater than its preset threshold value, then the corresponding flag, here **Flag$_{11}$**, is set to 1 otherwise it remains at 0. Table 10.2 is a signature table which includes the early possible signs leading to a fault. In order to decide on a fault, the algorithm makes a bit test with each sign. If the combination of detected flags matches the corresponding signature of a sign, it means that a fault has definitely 'occurred' in the system, otherwise it is a false alarm. The rules used for the test are simple (Isermann and Freyermuth, 1991):

IF (detected sign = signature) **THEN**

   fault type = sign #

Table 10.2   Binary code for early signs prior to a diagnosis: fault signatures

Sign	$\|Error_1\|$ Flag$_{11}$	$\|Error_2\|$ Flag$_{21}$	$\|Rate_1\|$ Flag$_{21}$	$\|Rate_2\|$ Flag$_{22}$	$Trace_1$ Flag$_{13}$	$Trace_2$ Flag$_{23}$
1	0	0	0	0	0	0
2	1	0	0	0	0	0
3	1	0	1	0	0	0
4	0	0	1	0	0	0
5	0	0	0	0	1	0
6	0	0	0	0	0	1
7	0	1	0	0	0	0
8	0	0	0	1	0	0

The nature of possible signs is outlined below:

- Sign 1: Sign of a slow drift. This could be an actuator fault but needs k samples to be sure. Also need to check that *Error* ≥ 0 and *Error rate* ≥ 0, and *input* $\neq 0$ for at least $(k - 1)$ samples.

- Sign 2: Patient movement that could be the result of a previous patient permanent movement, or the late stage of an actuator fault. This needs k samples to be sure.

- Sign 3: *Error* and *Error rate* beyond their respective thresholds. This is definitely a patient movement in the muscle relaxation channel. This needs k samples to show if it is a recoverable or a permanent one.

- Sign 4: *Error* is low but *Error rate* is high. This feature definitely characterises a sudden recoverable disturbance from a patient's arm movement or diathermy.

- Sign 5: Estimator 1 incorrectly learning the process.

- Sign 6: Estimator 2 incorrectly learning the process.

- Sign 7: *Error* and *Error rate* are beyond their respective thresholds. This is definitely a patient movement in the blood pressure channel. This needs k samples to show if it is a recoverable or a permanent one.

- Sign 8: *Error* is low but *Error rate* is high. This feature definitely characterises a sudden recoverable disturbance in the blood pressure channel.

Accommodation (compensation)

Once the source of the fault has been identified, accommodation or compensation must be provided. For a sudden disturbance, caused by either diathermy or a patient's arm movement, the use of an observer filter $T(z^{-1})$ together with the model-following polynomial $P(z^{-1})$ should suffice to reject it. However, for a patient permanent movement that is likely to last more than three samples, the idea of adapting the current set-point level to the new output indicated by the Relaxograph device seems to be one possible solution until the initial state is again recovered. As for the actuator's fault, the automatic control provided by GPC should be stopped, until the fault is repaired. If, however, the covariance trace of the ith estimator $(i = 1, 2)$ is too low, then a covariance resetting operation is one possible solution in order to restore the above estimator's integrity.

Finally, in the event of at least one of the closed-loop poles being found to lie outside the unit circle, the current control run is switched to a more conservative control (fixed GPC control) and the GPC tuning factors adjusted for better closed-loop regulation. This operation is carried out only in the transient stages (i.e. when the FDIA operations are disabled). To illustrate this consider the control system in the form of a pole placement problem.

Rewrite equation (2.20) explicitly as:

$$\Delta u(t) = [g_0, \ldots, g_{N_2-1}](\omega - \Psi) \tag{10.11}$$

The first incremental signal is obtained by combining the above equation with that of (2.14),

$$\Delta u(t) = \sum_{j=N_1}^{N_2} g_{j-1}\omega(t+j) - \sum_{j=N_1}^{N_2} h_j \frac{\bar{G}_j}{T} \Delta u(t-1) - \sum_{j=N_1}^{N_2} h_j \frac{F_j}{TP_d} y(t) \tag{10.12}$$

This then leads to the following control equation:

$$\left(TP_d + P_d \sum_{j=N_1}^{N_2} h_j \bar{G}_j z^{-1}\right)\Delta u(t) = \left(P_d \sum_{j=N_1}^{N_2} h_j z^{(-N_2+j)}\right)\omega(t + N_2) - \left(\sum_{j=N_1}^{N_2} h_j F_j\right)y(t)$$

(10.13)

The above equation is in the form of a pole-placement design problem and can be rewritten as the following:

$$K\Delta u(t) = TL\omega(t + N_2) - My(t)$$

(10.14)

Substituting equation (10.14) into the plant model (2.11) gives:

$$(KA\Delta + BMz^{-1})y(t) = BTL\omega(t + N_2 - 1) + KT\xi(t)$$

(10.15)

Now $(KA\Delta + BMz^{-1}) = 0$ is the closed-loop characteristic equation. Applying equations (2.15), (2.16) and (2.19) to equation (10.15) gives:

$$(KA\Delta + BMz^{-1}) = T\left[A\Delta P_d + \sum_{j=N_1}^{N_2} h_j(P_n B - A\Delta P_d \bar{\bar{G}})z^{(j-1)}\right] = TA_c$$

(10.16)

This leads therefore to the following controlled equation:

$$y(t) = B\frac{K}{A_c}\omega(t + N_2 - 1) + \frac{K}{A_c}\xi(t)$$

(10.17)

The problem of stability requires the solution of the roots of the closed-loop characteristic equation $A_c = 0$.

10.4   Simulation results

The simulation studies utilised the continuous anaesthetic model. A fourth-order Runge–Kutta method was used with a fixed step length of 0.1 and a sampling interval of 1 minute. For parameter estimation, a UD-factorisation method was used on incremental data with initial covariance matrix and forgetting factor given by: $Cov = 10^2.I$ and $\rho = 0.975$ respectively. In the multivariable GPC case, a multivariable model of 5 diagonal $A(z^{-1})$ matrices together with 5 upper triangular $B(z^{-1})$ matrices was estimated (see Chapter 4). In the GPCF case, however, a third-order model with a time delay of 1 minute and with two coefficients for the feedforward was considered for the first channel (muscle relaxation), while for the second channel (blood pressure) a first-order model also with a 1 minute time delay was considered (see Chapter 4). Initial conditions were 0% relaxation and 100 mmHg arterial pressure. The set-point command signal was 80% then 70% for relaxation, and 80 mmHg then 70 mmHg for the blood pressure. A bolus dose u_1 of atracurium of 67 mg at 1 mg ml^{-1} concentration was initially applied for one sample and input u_2 was kept at 0. While the bolus effect took place, the loop remained open until the output in the muscle relaxation channel reached the safety level of 85% when the loop was closed. The self-tuner was allowed to run with the initial parameter estimates until sample time 39 min (where a steady state can be considered to have been safely reached) at which time the parameter estimation routine was allowed to be operational. The FDIA scheme was allowed to be active from the sample time 64 min. All experiments were conducted over a fixed period of time of 300 minutes. The study was divided into two parts: the first part concerned the application of the GPCF algorithm, while the second considered the use of the multivariable version of the GPC algorithm together with a P-canonical form for the process model. In either case the adopted GPC tuning knobs were as follows:

$$N_1 = 1, \quad N_2 = 10, \quad NU(\text{ch } 1) = 2, \quad NU(\text{ch } 2) = 1,$$

$$P = \begin{bmatrix} \dfrac{(1 - 0.7z^{-1})}{0.3} & 0 \\[2mm] 0 & \dfrac{(1 - 0.9z^{-1})}{0.1} \end{bmatrix}$$

In the multivariable GPCF case:

$$T(z^{-1}) = \begin{cases} \begin{bmatrix} (1 - 0.8z^{-1})^2 & 0 \\ 0 & (1 - 0.85z^{-1})^2 \end{bmatrix} & \text{for control} \\[4mm] \begin{bmatrix} (1 - 0.8z^{-1})^2 & 0 \\ 0 & (1 - 0.85z^{-1})^2 \end{bmatrix} & \text{for estimation} \end{cases}$$

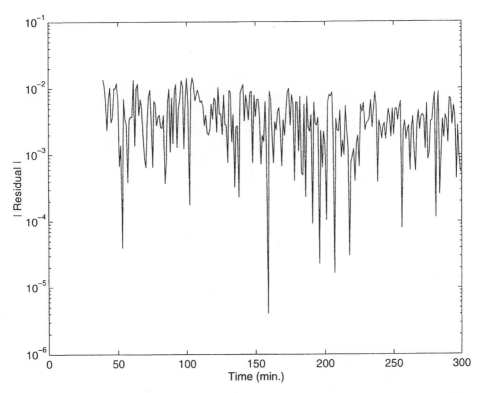

Figure 10.5 Recorded prediction error values in the noisy case for channel 1 in the multivariable GPCF case.

In the multivariable GPC case:

$$
T(z^{-1}) = \begin{cases} \begin{bmatrix} (1 - 0.8z^{-1})^2 & 0 \\ 0 & (1 - 0.8z^{-1})^2 \end{bmatrix} & \text{for control} \\ \begin{bmatrix} (1 - 0.8z^{-1})^2 & 0 \\ 0 & (1 - 0.85z^{-1})^2 \end{bmatrix} & \text{for estimation} \end{cases}
$$

At this stage it is also worth noting that the set-point profile was pre-specified to the GPC algorithm ten samples in advance, this having the effect of reducing the interaction in the muscle relaxation loop (see Chapter 9). However, before describing the experiments carried out in this simulation study it is worth reviewing the procedure adopted for determining the thresholds necessary for detection and diagnosis.

10.4.1   Determination of residuals' and signals' thresholds

The normal procedure adopted in this case is to gather enough information on the normal operating conditions of the system, i.e. under fault-free conditions. In light of these considerations, a simulation study was conducted in which the residual in the muscle relaxation channel was recorded for a period of 300 minutes under the above assumed conditions. The results are shown in Figures 10.5 and 10.6, where the absolute values of the prediction error are plotted against time on a semi-

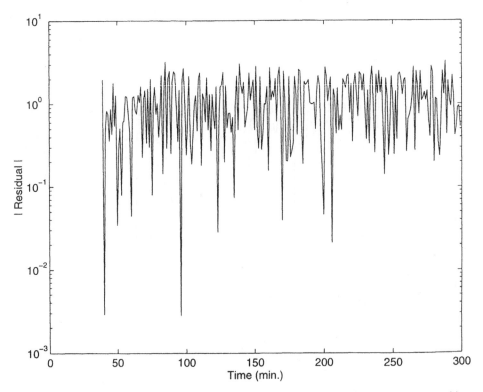

Figure 10.6   Recorded prediction error values in the noisy case for channel 2 in the multivariable GPCF case.

logarithmic scale (under noisy conditions). Similar tests were performed under noise-free conditions. Hence, for the two channels the absolute values of the residual thresholds were chosen to be as follows.

- For channel 1:

$$J_{thr} \begin{cases} 3 \cdot 10^{-3} & \text{for a noise-free environment} \\ 10^{-2} & \text{for a noisy environment} \end{cases} \tag{10.18}$$

- For channel 2

$$J_{thr} = \begin{cases} 1.0 & \text{for a noise-free environment} \\ 4.0 & \text{for a noisy environment} \end{cases} \tag{10.19}$$

For the thresholds relating to $|Error|$ and $|Error\ rate|$ the following quantities were adopted for the two categories 'low' and 'high' throughout:

- For channel 1:

$$\begin{aligned} \text{Low:} \quad & 0.0 \leq |Error| < 0.05 \\ \text{High:} \quad & |Error| \geq 0.05 \end{aligned} \tag{10.20}$$

$$\begin{aligned} \text{Low:} \quad & 0.0 \leq |Error\ rate| < 0.05 \\ \text{High:} \quad & |Error\ rate| \geq 0.05 \end{aligned} \tag{10.21}$$

- For channel 2:

$$\begin{aligned} \text{Low:} \quad & 0.0 \leq |Error| < 5.5 \\ \text{High:} \quad & |Error| \geq 5.5 \end{aligned} \tag{10.22}$$

$$\begin{aligned} \text{Low:} \quad & 0.0 \leq |Error\ rate| < 5.5 \\ \text{High:} \quad & |Error\ rate| \geq 5.5 \end{aligned} \tag{10.23}$$

The results are divided into two parts, the first part being concerned with the performance of the gain scheduling block, whereas the second deals with the performance of the remaining blocks in the hierarchical supervisory layer.

10.4.2   Results of experiments

Performance of the gain scheduling block

Varying the patient's gain to atracurium between 1 and 3 and applying different bolus doses over a 1 minute period in each case produced the results of Table 10.3 which show the estimated gain in each case to be close to the true value.

Table 10.3 Performance of the gain scheduling block in estimating the patient's gain to a single bolus dose of atracurium

True gain	Bolus size (mg)	Output magnitude	Peak time (min)	Estimated gain
1.0	67	0.9754	6.0	1.01
2.0	42	0.9872	6.0	2.02
3.0	42	0.9961	6.0	3.03

In order to estimate a patient's gain to isoflurane, a 1% step change in isoflurane was applied to the first-order process over a 25 minute sample, while a noise sequence of amplitude 2.5 mmHg was superimposed on the output. The true process gain was taken to be -15.0. The data points obtained were then filtered using a median filter (Heinonen and Neuvo, 1987). The final patient's gain to isoflurane can be obtained by taking the average of the last few points for instance. In this case, for a 3 point averaging filter the estimated gain was approximately -14.77.

Performance of the FDIA block under the multivariable GPCF algorithm

Fault-free case For the above conditions for the estimator and the controller a run was conducted using the GPCF control strategy. The result is shown in Figure 10.7 where the performance was good with minimum interactions in the muscle relaxation channel despite the set-point changes in the blood pressure channel. Figure 10.8 also shows a good performance and a reasonably active signal when noise sequences were superimposed on the various outputs of the process ($\pm 0.5\%$ for channel 1 and ± 2.5 mmHg for channel 2).

Faulty conditions case First, a sudden recoverable output disturbance of 6% in channel 1 was simulated at sample time 70 min (see Figure 10.9). As the on-line screendump of Figure 10.10 shows that the algorithm detected the fault and diagnosed it as a recoverable one and assumed that the filter polynomial $T(z^{-1})$ would reject it. Hence, no further action was taken as a result (the first two binary numbers of

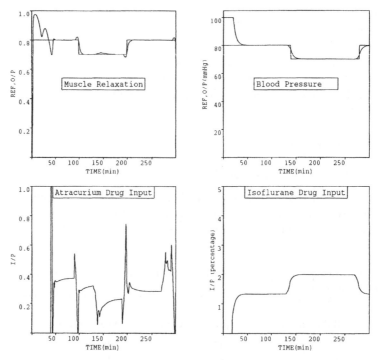

Figure 10.7 Adaptive control of the anaesthetic model in a fault-free environment; multivariable GPCF algorithm, noise-free environment.

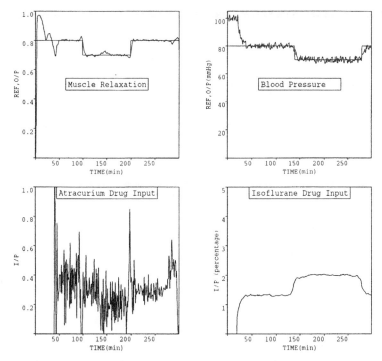

Figure 10.8 Adaptive control of the anaesthetic model in a fault-free environment; multivariable GPCF algorithm, noisy environment.

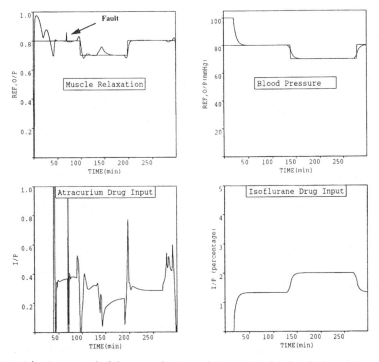

Figure 10.9 Adaptive control of the anaesthetic model in a noise-free but faulty environment; (6% disturbance in channel 1), multivariable GPCF algorithm.

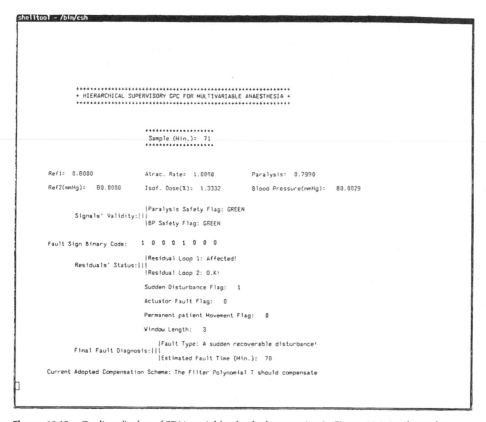

Figure 10.10   On-line display of FDIA variables for fault occurring in Figure 10.9 (in channel 1).

the fault sign binary code represent the flag settings relating to the prediction errors in the respective channels: 0 if O.K. and 1 if affected, the rest of the code is as outlined in Table 10.2). Figure 10.11 represents the variations of the absolute values of the prediction error, relative to the channel affected, against time. The overall performance obtained can be judged as good despite the set-point change which occurred shortly after the fault.

The second experiment consisted of simulating a permanent shift in the paralysis level at sample time 70 min (under noisy conditions) which lasted until sample time 198 min as demonstrated in Figure 10.12. The on-line screendump of Figure 10.13 shows that the algorithm recognised the fault as being a non-recoverable shift in the paralysis level and compensated for it by adapting the actual set-point to the first recorded output value which was 0.72. Figure 10.14 also shows that when the paralysis recovered its initial state the algorithm recognised this as a fault and adapted the set-point to the new current output value 0.80.

Performance of the FDIA block under the multivariable GPC algorithm

Fault-free case   Repeating the same procedure as above, the runs produced the output responses of Figures 10.15 and 10.16 where it can be seen that the performances were good with minimum interactions from the blood pressure channel. This is

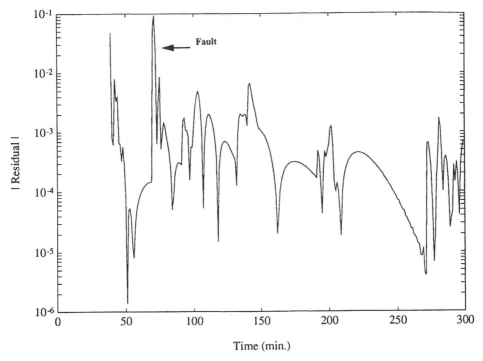

Figure 10.11   Recorded prediction-error values corresponding to Figure 10.9.

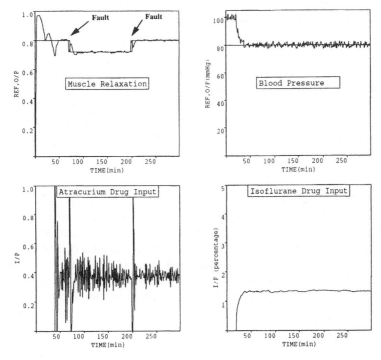

Figure 10.12   Adaptive control of the anaesthetic model in a noisy and faulty environment; (permanent patient movement in channel 1), multivariable GPCF algorithm.

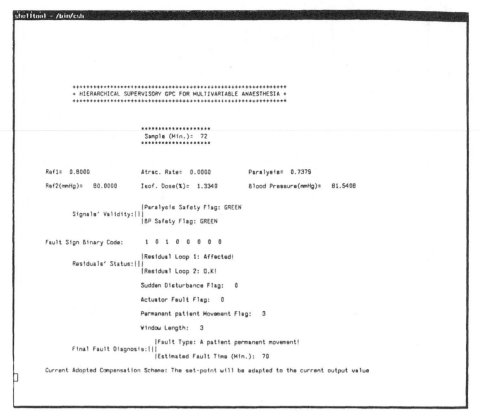

Figure 10.13   On-line display of FDIA variables for first fault occurring in Figure 10.12.

perhaps due to the fact that the pre-specified set-point approach works better with the full multivariable concept than with the SISO approach.

Faulty conditions case   A sudden output disturbance of 7 mmHg was simulated in the blood pressure channel at sample time 170 min and under noise-free conditions. The FDIA block detected this as being a recoverable disturbance and left the filter polynomial to compensate for it as clearly shown in Figure 10.17. Finally, a malfunction of the syringe pump unit in channel 1 was simulated at sample time 70 min under noise-corrupted conditions. Here again, the FDIA block set the right flag to the window length, indicating that there was indeed a malfunction of the pump as shown in Figures 10.18 and 10.19. A complete shut-down operation was executed in this case. Notice that the estimated fault time is three samples behind the true time occurrence of the fault (one sample due to the transport delay and two samples due to the appearance of the fault in the actual data which were corrupted by noise) implying that the fault symptoms are normally delayed by this amount.

10.5   Conclusions

The growing demand for fault tolerance in control systems has been prompted by the advances made in automatic control as well as those in computer technology

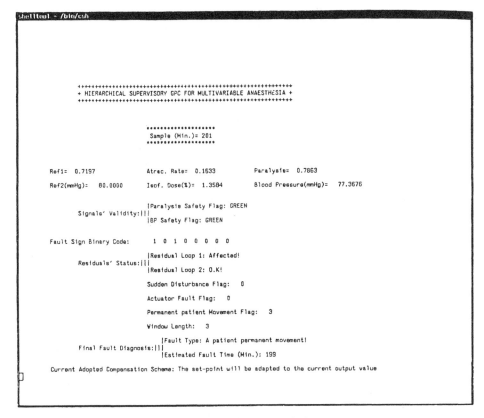

Figure 10.14 On-line display of FDIA variables for second fault occurring in Figure 10.12.

which have led to the possibility of obtaining high systems performances in relatively short time scales. Biomedicine, being such a sensitive area, is among the later areas to be associated with this form of control requiring demonstration that it is safe and effective not only on animals but also on humans. Self-adaptive GPC has been applied successfully in theatre with little interaction being required by the anaesthetist, and the multivariable version of the same control strategy applied to a multivariable model of anaesthesia has been the subject of a detailed study presented in chapter 4. In this chapter it has been shown that an intelligent structure can be given to the existing algorithm by adding a supervisory layer that monitors the variables involved and assesses the performance of the overall control system. By doing this, the controller is able to fulfil three tasks successfully, namely: control, adaptation and supervision.

The study saw the application of two strategies stemming from the same algorithm, i.e. multivariable GPC using a P-canonical form together with a triangular structure for the $B(z^{-1})$ matrices, and the GPCF algorithm. In principle, the two approaches can be considered as equivalent since it is widely known that the P-canonical form considers these interactions as feedforward terms, although the number of estimated parameters in this case is far greater than in the GPCF case. In formulation, however, they differ slightly since in the GPCF case future control increments from the interacting channel are considered to be zero as already outlined in the previous sections. Also, because the multivariable GPCF algorithm

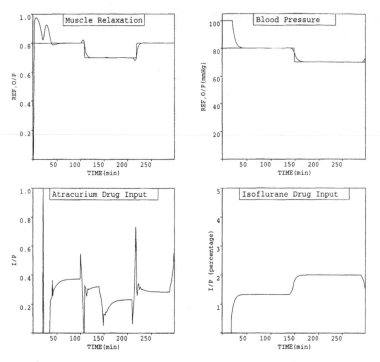

Figure 10.15 Adaptive control of the anaesthetic model in a fault-free environment; multivariable GPC algorithm, noise-free environment.

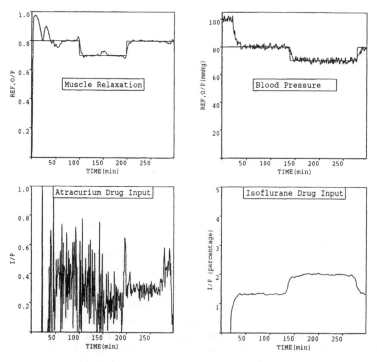

Figure 10.16 Adaptive control of the anaesthetic model in a fault-free environment; multivariable GPC algorithm, noisy environment.

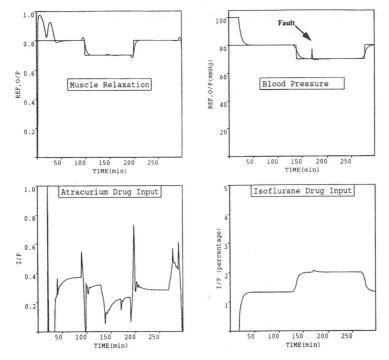

Figure 10.17   Adaptive control of the anaesthetic model in a noise-free but faulty environment; (7 mmHg disturbance in channel 2), multivariable GPC algorithm.

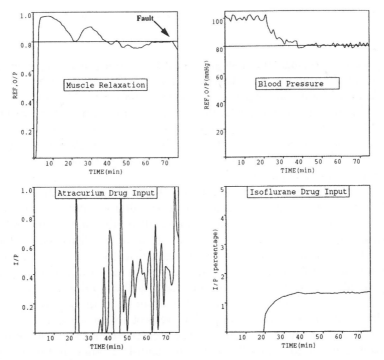

Figure 10.18   Adaptive control of the anaesthetic model in a noisy and faulty environment; (malfunction of the syringe pump in channel 1), multivariable GPC algorithm.

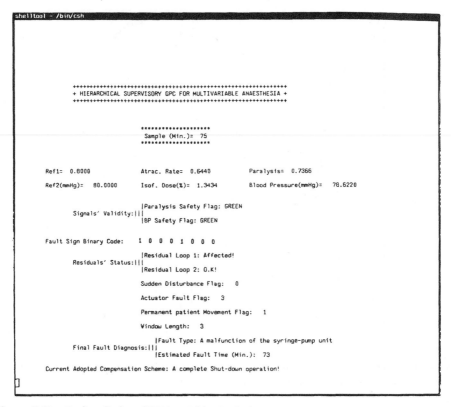

```
shelltool - /bin/csh


         ++++++++++++++++++++++++++++++++++++++++++++++++++++++++++
         + HIERARCHICAL SUPERVISORY GPC FOR MULTIVARIABLE ANAESTHESIA +
         ++++++++++++++++++++++++++++++++++++++++++++++++++++++++++


                    ********************
                    Sample (Min.)=  75
                    ********************


    Ref1=  0.8000          Atrac. Rate=  0.6440          Paralysis=  0.7366

    Ref2(mmHg)=  80.0000   Isof. Dose(%)=  1.3434        Blood Pressure(mmHg)=   78.6220

                           |Paralysis Safety Flag: GREEN
            Signals' Validity:|||
                           |BP Safety Flag: GREEN


    Fault Sign Binary Code:   1  0  0  0  1  0  0  0

                           |Residual Loop 1: Affected!
            Residuals' Status:|||
                           |Residual Loop 2: O.K!

                    Sudden Disturbance Flag:   0

                    Actuator Fault Flag:   3

                    Permanent patient Movement Flag:   1

                    Window Length:   3

                           |Fault Type: A malfunction of the syringe-pump unit
            Final Fault Diagnosis:|||
                           |Estimated Fault Time (Min.):  73

    Current Adopted Compensation Scheme: A complete Shut-down operation!
```

Figure 10.19   On-line display of FDIA variables for fault occurring in Figure 10.18.

consists of only two single-input single-output GPC loops linked by a feedforward term, it is more attractive than the multivariable GPC algorithm as far as calculating the closed-loop characteristic equations is concerned. Moreover, it must be said that although the performances that were obtained with both algorithms were comparable, the control signal generated in the muscle relaxation channel in the presence of noise was less active in the multivariable GPCF case than in the multivariable GPC case due to the lower number of estimated parameters subject to uncertainty (see also Chapter 6).

The use of bolus injections in the initial stages of the experiment could have made the estimator's job more difficult since it was disabled during that period, but the gain scheduling block whose task was to evaluate the gains in the main loops, demonstrated that it can infer these values quite accurately. This enables the multivariable GPC algorithm to regulate the process efficiently when it is used in a fixed mode, until reasonable data can be gathered from within the closed-loop prior to the start of adaptation. For detection, the use of a P-canonical form in the multivariable model as well as the feedforward philosophy in the multivariable GPCF case, helps to decouple the two loops with respect to checking the two different prediction errors for faults. The thresholds for determining the existence of a fault had to be determined from an off-line run in a fault-free situation. For all the faults considered, which featured two abrupt changes and one slow drift, the prediction error evaluation provided an effective source of fault detection. The faults isolation or diagnosis, whose philosophy stems from several authors' suggestions (Isermann, 1981, 1984; Beneken and Gravenstein, 1987; Blom *et al.*, 1985), i.e. the use of absolute signals and their trends, was also effective in 'pin-pointing' a particular fault type inferred from a catalogue of 'could-be' faults. For one type of these faults (a sudden recoverable disturbance) the inherent structure of the GPC strategy allows automatic compensation by inclusion of the observer polynomial $T(z^{-1})$ providing that its characteristics are adequately chosen. The results obtained with both strategies are very encouraging, and it is hoped to develop the system further with respect to faults relating to the patients' metabolism such as blood loss, large fluctuations in cardiac ouput and other emergency conditions normally encountered during a surgical operation.

CHAPTER ELEVEN

Nonlinear Generalised Predictive Control (NLGPC) for Muscle Relaxant Anaesthesia

11.1 Introduction

As already mentioned in the previous chapters, the theme of model-based predictive control (MBPC) and particularly that of GPC has been developed extensively to deal with various system complexities such as large dead-times, instability, unmodelled dynamics, etc. This has been achieved by means of formulation of a linearised model of the system in question, severe nonlinearities being tackled by assuming that the system is linear around some operating point. By doing this, GPC has offered alternative design methods to well-known approaches such as fuzzy logic theory or neural networks. The bottleneck in any self-tuning adaptive control technique is the parameter estimation it uses. The estimation of a linear system is a straightforward operation practically, once a model structure is decided upon. However, if it is wished to estimate a nonlinear structure, the problem becomes more complicated. In MBPC, efforts have been made at devising self-tuning controllers for particular classes of nonlinear systems. Early work on nonlinear self-tuning control can be attributed to Agarwal and Seborg (1987) who devised a nonlinear version of the generalised minimum variance (GMV) controller. As far as long range predictive control is concerned, Bars and Haber (1988, 1991) developed controllers for nonlinear systems represented by Volterra series whose parameters can be estimated by an extended recursive least-squares algorithm with scalar convergence coefficients such as the Kaczmarcz algorithm. An adaptive GPC controller for systems which can be described by a Hammerstein model was also proposed by Warwick *et al.* (1991); the nonlinear and linear parts are treated separately and here too the model parameters are estimated using an extended least-squares estimation algorithm similar to that proposed by Kortmann and Unbehauen (1987). In the research work presented in this chapter a nonlinear GPC controller is proposed for muscle relaxant anaesthesia which can be modelled, as we have already seen in Chapter 2, by a Wiener structure; a linear part which includes a third-order transfer function with dead-time and transmission zero followed by a severe nonlinear part

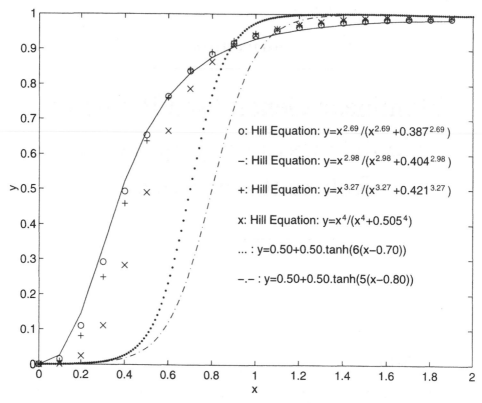

Figure 11.1 Graph showing the shape of the various nonlinearity curves used in the system and model.

in the shape of a Hill equation (sigmoidal function). Clinical results in operating theatre involving the use of GPC based on the linearised model have already been described in Chapter 2 with targets close to 15%, in contrast to the technique presented in this chapter which takes into account the nonlinear predictions of the process outputs some horizons ahead. The new controller's benefits are apparent when the regulation is chosen to be close to the saturation zone (up to 5% EMG targets), a very challenging task due to the difficulty of saturation nonlinearity in the muscle relaxation sigmoid, and also when the time delay is large (Agarwal and Seborg, 1987).

Recall the mathematical model associated with the drug atracurium and which was described by equation (2.8):

$$\frac{V(s)}{U(s)} = \frac{1.5(1 + 10.6s)\,e^{-s}}{(1 + 34.4s)(1 + 4.8s)(1 + 3.1s)} \tag{11.1}$$

and the overall nonlinear model is obtained by combining equation (11.1) together with the Hill equation already described by equation (2.7), i.e.

$$\begin{cases} Y = \dfrac{V^\alpha}{(V^\alpha + V^\alpha_{50})} \\ \alpha = 2.98 \pm 0.29 \\ v_{50} = 0.404 \pm 0.017 \end{cases} \qquad (11.2)$$

Figure 11.1 shows a series of curves represented by the Hill equation for different parameters of α and v_{50}, as well as another type of nonlinearity which will be described in later sections. Notice that for nominal Hill equation values, a linearised gain for operating points ranging from 0.85 to 0.95 for paralysis can lead to difficulties due to the curved shape around this region. Also, the patient-to-patient parameter variability can affect the nonlinearity shape by making it steeper or more flat. Hence, all these considerations make the muscle relaxation process a very challenging one.

11.2 Theory of the proposed nonlinear GPC algorithm (NLGPC)

A block diagram of the specific nonlinear controller based on the generalised predictive control (GPC) algorithm is shown in Figure 11.2. The idea behind this controller is as follows: at each sampling time, a nonlinear signal $y(t)$ is obtained and a linear signal $v(t)$ is inferred using an assumed inverse model of the nonlinearity which is represented by a Hill equation (the signal $v(t)$ which is equivalent to a blood concentration is not a measurable signal). This signal together with the input signal $u(t)$ are used to identify the assumed linear part of the model. In turn, the obtained parameter estimates are used to predict the future linear signals of $v(t)$ (i.e. $v(t + 1)$, $v(t + 2)$, ...), and with these predicted outputs the relationship between $v(t)$ and $y(t)$ is used to predict the future nonlinear signals of $y(t)$ (i.e. $y(t + 1)$, $y(t + 2)$, ...). The GPC cost function is formed and the solution $\tilde{u}$ is obtained by minimisation of this cost function using techniques such as genetic algorithms as will be explained later. The following is a description of the above strategy.

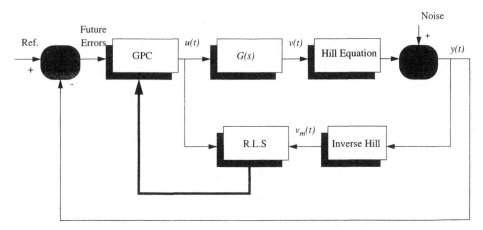

Figure 11.2 Schematic diagram depicting the structure of the nonlinear GPC controller.

Taking into account the diagram of Figure 11.2 and using GPC's strategy, the future output signals of the linear part can be written as follows:

$$
\begin{cases}
\hat{v}_m(t+1) = g_0\,\Delta u(t) + f(t+1) \\
\hat{v}_m(t+2) = g_1\Delta u(t) + g_0\,\Delta u(t+1) + f(t+2) \\
\;\;\vdots \\
\hat{v}_m(t+N_2) = g_{(N_2-1)}\,\Delta u(t) + \ldots + g_{(N_2-NU)}\Delta u(t+N_2-NU) + f(t+N_2)
\end{cases}
\tag{11.3}
$$

where according to equation (2.14):

$$
\begin{cases}
f(t+j) = \bar{G}_j\,\Delta u^f(t-1) + F_j\hat{v}_m^f(t) \\
v_m(t) = D_m\!\left(\dfrac{y}{(1-y)}\right)^{1/\alpha_m}
\end{cases}
\tag{11.4}
$$

α_m and D_m represent the assumed model parameters of the Hill equation. Hence, the nonlinear signal $y(t)$ can be written as follows:

$$
y(t) = \frac{v(t)^{\alpha_m}}{(v(t)^{\alpha_m} + D_m^{\alpha_m})}
\tag{11.5}
$$

Using the following properties of the backward shift operator z:

$$
\begin{aligned}
z^j\phi(t) &= \phi(t+j) \\
z^j[\phi(t)\psi(t)] &= \phi(t+j)\psi(t+j)
\end{aligned}
\tag{11.6}
$$

one can write the predicted nonlinear signals $\hat{y}(t+j)$ as follows:

$$
\begin{cases}
\hat{y}(t+1) = \dfrac{\hat{v}_m(t+1)^{\alpha_m}}{(\hat{v}_m(t+1)^{\alpha_m} + D_m^{\alpha_m})} \\[2mm]
\hat{y}(t+2) = \dfrac{\hat{v}_m(t+2)^{\alpha_m}}{(\hat{v}_m(t+2)^{\alpha_m} + D_m^{\alpha_m})} \\[1mm]
\;\;\vdots \\[1mm]
\hat{y}(t+N_2) = \dfrac{\hat{v}_m(t+N_2)^{\alpha_m}}{(\hat{v}_m(t+N_2)^{\alpha_m} + D_m^{\alpha_m})}
\end{cases}
\tag{11.7}
$$

The signals $\hat{v}(t+j)$, $j = 1, 2, \ldots, N_2$ are the ones predicted by the linear GPC controller according to equation (11.3).

The cost function (2.12) to be optimised is reformulated as the following:

$$
\left\{ J_{nl} = \sum_{j=N_1}^{N_2}\left[(\hat{y}(t+j) - \omega(t+j))^2\right] + \sum_{j=1}^{NU}[\lambda(j)(\Delta u(t+j-1))^2]
\tag{11.8}
\right.
$$

This function being no longer differentiable, a solution using numerical optimisation methods such as the golden section search method for $NU = 1$, the modified simplex method of Nelder–Mead when $NU > 1$ or genetic algorithms can be used, as will be demonstrated in the next section which is concerned with the simulation results.

11.3   Simulation results

The simulation studies utilised the continuous muscle relaxation model described by equations (11.1) and (11.2). A fourth-order Runge–Kutta method was used with a fixed step length of 0.1 and a sampling interval of 1 minute. For parameter estimation a UD-factorisation method was used on incremental data with initial covariance matrix and forgetting factor given by: $Cov = 10^3 . I$ and $\rho = 0.97$ respectively. This was triggered at the same time as closed-loop control was established with the first b parameter initialised to a value of 1. A third-order model of 3 as and 3 bs was estimated with an assumed time delay of 1 minute. Initial conditions were 0% relaxation. The set-point command signal was 0.80 (20% EMG) for the first 100 minutes, 0.95 (5% EMG) for the next 100 minutes, 0.90 (10% EMG) for a further 50 minutes, and finally 0.95 (5% EMG) until the end of the simulation. The control signal was clipped between 0 and 1.

In order to minimise equation (11.8), three methods were used: the golden section search method (when $NU = 1$) (Rao, 1984), the popular genetic algorithms (when $NU = 1$) (Goldberg, 1989), and the modified simplex method of Nelder–Mead (when $NU > 1$) (Fletcher, 1980). The experiments were divided into three categories: the first category comprised the linearised controller, the second category comprised the nonlinear GPC when the nonlinearity structure in the system matched that assumed in the model, and the third category comprised experiments when a structure mismatch between the assumed model and the actual system was considered.

11.3.1   The standard linear GPC algorithm

First, the linear GPC controller described by equation (2.20) was considered. A combination of (1, 10, 1, 0) was assumed for (N_1, N_2, NU, λ), and an observer polynomial of $T(z^{-1}) = (1 - 0.8\, z^{-1})^2$ was also used for estimation (with incremental data) and control. The linear GPC led to the performance of Figure 11.3 where the controller found it hard to settle initially because of saturation of the input signal, and at the higher set-point of 0.95 the input signal was too sluggish rendering the output unable to track the set-point fast enough. When the control horizon was increased to 2, hence increasing the controller's degrees of freedom, the performance obtained was that of Figure 11.4 which shows a more active signal initially which led to the poor transient followed by a control signal with ripples. When a noise sequence was superimposed on the output, the experiment led to Figure 11.5 which displayed a highly active control signal despite the inclusion of the above observer polynomial. However, such control activity can be reduced by the inclusion of the weighting sequence λ, as shown in Figure 11.6, at the expense of a slower output tracking response.

11.3.2   Nonlinear GPC with matched nonlinear structure

Solution using classical numerical optimisation methods

The nonlinear GPC described by equations (11.3)–(11.8) was implemented and the minimisation of equation (11.8) was achieved using the golden section search

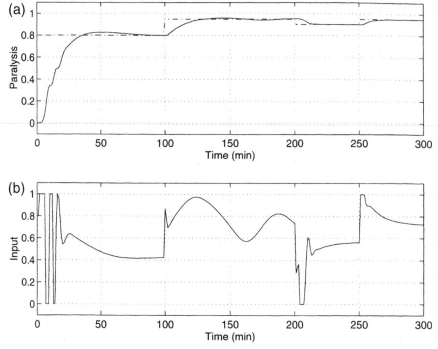

Figure 11.3 Linear GPC of muscle relaxation; $NU = 1$, $T(z^{-1}) = (1 - 0.8z^{-1})^2$. (a) Solid line: paralysis; dashdot line: target. (b) Input signal.

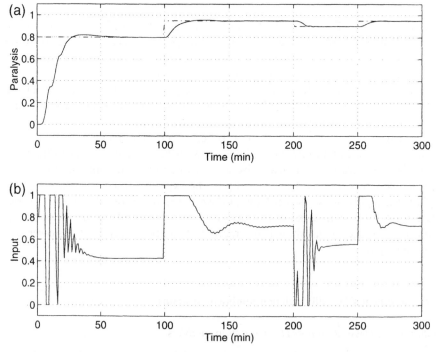

Figure 11.4 Linear GPC of muscle relaxation; $NU = 2$, $T(z^{-1}) = (1 - 0.8z^{-1})^2$. (a) Solid line: paralysis; dashdot line: target. (b) Input signal.

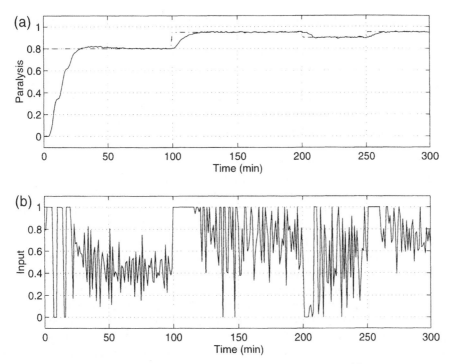

Figure 11.5 Linear GPC of muscle relaxation; $NU = 2$, $T(z^{-1}) = (1 - 0.8z^{-1})^2$ with additive output noise. (a) Solid line: paralysis; dashdot line: target. (b) Input signal.

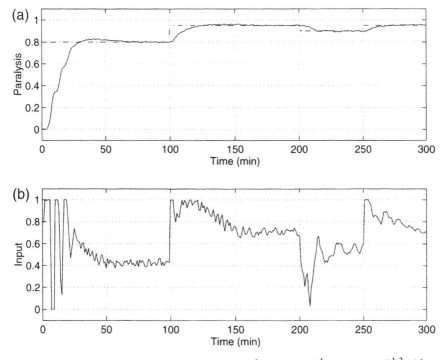

Figure 11.6 Linear GPC of muscle relaxation; $NU = 2$, $\lambda = 0.01$, $T(z^{-1}) = (1 - 0.8z^{-1})^2$ with additive output noise. (a) Solid line: paralysis; dashdot line: target. (b) Input signal.

method when $NU = 1$ and the modified simplex method of Nelder–Mead when $NU \geq 2$.

When $NU = 1$, the nonlinear GPC algorithm led to the performance of Figure 11.7 which, compared to that of Figure 11.3, has significantly better properties in terms of response speed and control signal activity. Figure 11.8 shows the surface generated by the functions (11.8) for the first 20 minutes indicating that as time progresses the parameter estimates improve which in turn produce a well-behaved surface. Increasing the control horizon to $NU = 2$ in the deterministic case led to the performance of Figure 11.9 where it can be seen that the control signal is considerably less active than that of Figure 11.4. In turn, when a noise sequence was added to the output, the controller's performance was good, as shown in Figure 11.10, with the output tracking the set-point efficiently and with a control signal much less active than that of Figure 11.5. The use of a weighting sequence of 0.01 led to the superior performance of Figure 11.11 without the loss of performance as incurred by the linear GPC (see Figure 11.6).

The robustness of the controller was also explored when a mismatch between the actual system's nonlinearity parameters and those of the model occurs. In our view this gives more credibility to the controller since it is only the linear part which is being estimated. Hence, the model assumed a nonlinearity described by $\alpha_m = 4.0$ and $D_m = 0.505$, whereas the system had the nominal parameters of equation (11.2) (see Figure 11.1 for amount of mismatch). The result of the run with $NU = 1$ is shown in Figure 11.12 where it can be seen that the controller coped very well

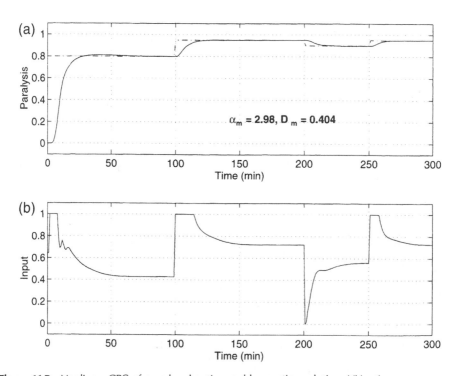

Figure 11.7   Nonlinear GPC of muscle relaxation; golden section solution, $NU = 1$, $T(z^{-1}) = (1 - 0.8z^{-1})^2$. (a) Solid line: paralysis; dashdot line: target. (b) Input signal.

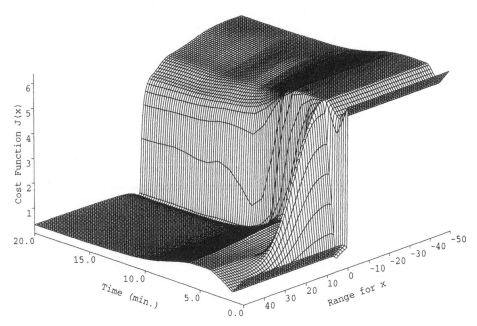

Figure 11.8   Three-dimensional representation of the cost functions for the first 20 minutes corresponding to the run of Figure 11.7a.

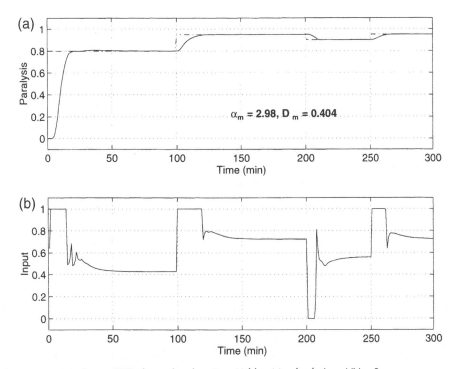

Figure 11.9   Nonlinear GPC of muscle relaxation; Nelder–Mead solution, $NU = 2$, $T(z^{-1}) = (1 - 0.8z^{-1})^2$. (a) Solid line: paralysis; dashdot line: target. (b) Input signal.

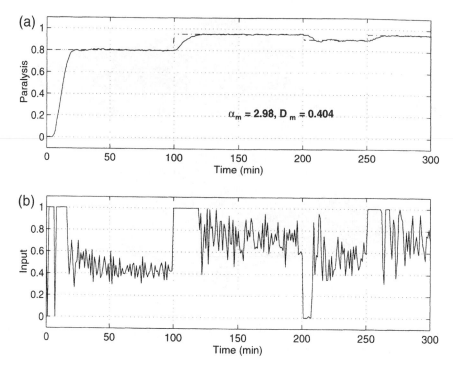

Figure 11.10   Nonlinear GPC of muscle relaxation; Nelder–Mead solution, $NU = 2$, $T(z^{-1}) = (1 - 0.8z^{-1})^2$ with additive output noise. (a) Solid line: paralysis; dashdot line: target. (b) Input signal.

without losing any of the previous characteristics, i.e. reasonable control activity and good set-point tracking ability.

Solution using genetic algorithms (GA)

The objective of this section is to show that the solution of the minimisation problem need not be confined to classical numerical methods, but instead can be obtained using other tools such as genetic algorithms (GA) (Goldberg, 1989).

Genetic algorithms are exploratory search and optimisation procedures that were devised on the principles of natural evolution and population genetics. First developed by Holland (1973, 1975), they combine survival of the fittest among string structures with a structured information exchange to form an efficient search algorithm which is in itself not random. Unlike other optimisation techniques, genetic algorithms do not require mathematical descriptions of the optimisation problem, but instead they rely on a cost function in order to assess the **fitness** of a particular solution to the problem in question. Possible solution candidates are represented by a **population** of individuals (**generation**) and each individual is encoded as a binary string containing a well-defined number of **chromosomes** (1s and 0s). Initially, a population of individuals is generated and the fittest individuals are chosen by ranking them according to an *a priori* defined fitness function which is evaluated for each member of this population. In order to create better generation from the initial one, a mating process is carried out among the fittest individuals in the previous

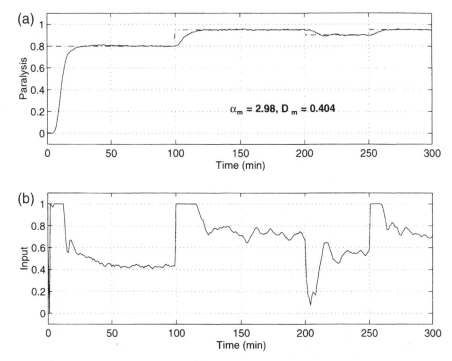

Figure 11.11 Nonlinear GPC of muscle relaxation; Nelder–Mead solution, $NU = 2$, $\lambda = 0.01$, $T(z^{-1}) = (1 - 0.8z^{-1})^2$ with additive output noise. (a) Solid line: paralysis; dashdot line: target. (b) Input signal.

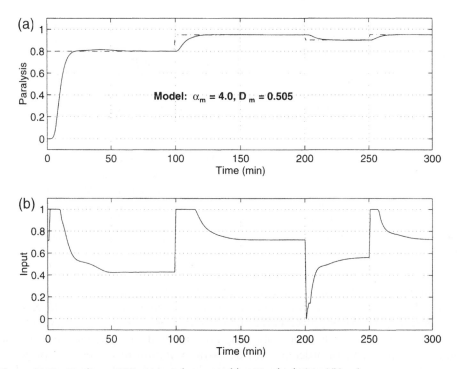

Figure 11.12 Nonlinear GPC; mismatch case, Nelder–Mead solution, $NU = 1$, $T(z^{-1}) = (1 - 0.8z^{-1})^2$. (a) Solid line: paralysis; dashdot line: target. (b) Input signal.

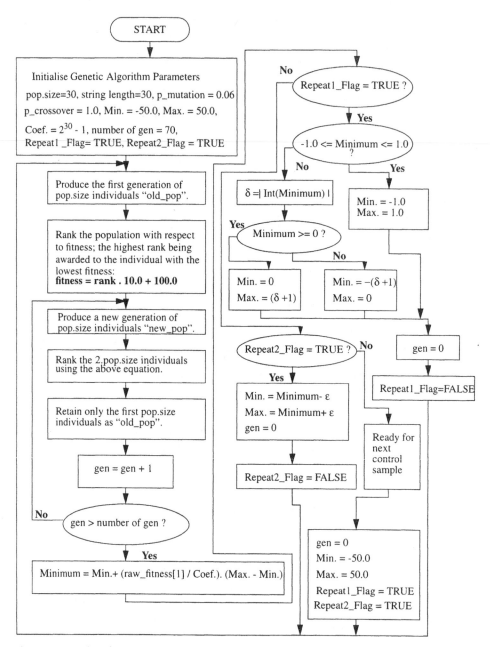

Figure 11.13 Flowchart representing the steps included in the genetic algorithm for solving equation (11.8).

generation, since the relative fitness of each individual is used as a criterion for choice. Hence, the selected individuals are randomly combined in pairs to produce two **offspring** by crossing over parts of their chromosomes at a randomly chosen position in the string. These new offspring are supposed to represent a better solution to the problem. In order to provide extra excitation to the process of generation, randomly chosen bits in the strings are inverted (0s to 1s and 1s to 0s). This mechanism is known as **mutation** and helps to speed up convergence and prevents the population from being predominated by the same individuals. A compromise, however, should be reached between too much excitation and none by choosing a small probability of mutation.

It is worth noting that many of the above-mentioned parameters are problem-related and one can only rely on guidelines for their choice. For instance, the process of creating generations can be allowed to operate for a predefined number of generations, or a tolerance for the fitness value can be set, this usually ensures that only the fittest individuals will survive within the final population. Hence, this technique has proved particularly useful in avoiding local minima which has been the underlying problem for most known numerical techniques.

In light of these considerations and to show that GAs can be used effectively in this instance, the experiment of Figure 11.7 was repeated using a GA with the following parameters:

Population size = 30

Chromosomes = 30

Probability of crossover = 1.0

Probability of mutation = 0.06

Number of generations = 70

Fitness scaling = $10 \times$ fitness rank + 100

Initial search interval = $[-50, 50]$

As far as breeding is concerned, the selective breeding method (Linkens and Nyongesa, 1995) was used. Initial simulation experiments suggested that with such a large initial search interval, the precision on the found minimum is poor, especially if the minimum is close to zero. Hence, in order to improve on this precision, the algorithm was modified according to the flowchart of Figure 11.13 where the interval is shrunk twice after an initial search in the interval $[-50, 50]$; the choice of the interval $[-1, 1]$ for the control increment $\Delta u(t)$ is justified by the physical constraints of the system itself, i.e. the control $u(t)$ is clipped within the interval $[0, 1]$. With this approach, using the selective breeding method, the performance of Figure 11.14, with $NU = 1$, was obtained and this is the same response as that of Figure 11.7.

11.3.3   Nonlinear GPC with a structural nonlinearity mismatch

At a control design stage, control engineers are normally expected to conduct a structural identification study to have an idea of the complexity of the system under investigation. Such a study allows the engineer to design a simulation platform under which the controller's robustness is tested before being transferred into the real application, in our case the operating theatre (see Chapters 2 and 4). Hence, in most cases the basic structure of the nonlinearity can be known. However, various structures may lead to roughly the same nonlinear effect (see Figure 11.1). In relaxant physiology, there is great uncertainty in structure and the Hill equation (11.2) represents only one hypothesis. In light of these considerations, and in order to

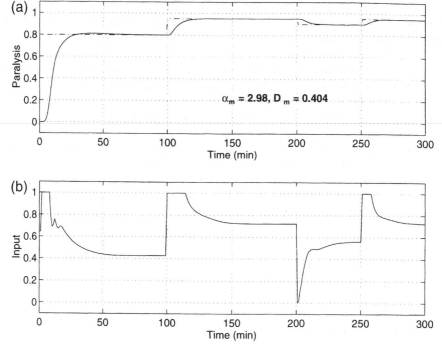

Figure 11.14 Nonlinear GPC; genetic algorithm solution, $NU = 1$, $T(z^{-1}) = (1 - 0.8z^{-1})^2$. (a) Solid line: paralysis; dashdot line: target. (b) Input signal.

assess the performance of the new controller, a scheme by which the linear signal $v_m(t)$ is obtained using a different nonlinearity pharmacodynamic structure proposed by Meager *et al.* (1989) was considered. The nonlinearity in this case is described by:

$$y(t) = y_0 + \gamma_0 \tanh(\beta(v(t) - v_0)) \tag{11.9}$$

In this particular case, the signal $v_m(t)$ can be inferred by the following formula:

$$v_m(t) = v_0 + \left(\frac{1}{\beta}\right)\tanh^{-1}\left[\frac{y(t) - y_0}{\gamma_0}\right]$$

$$\tanh^{-1}(x) = \log\left(\frac{1 + x}{1 - x}\right)^{1/2} \tag{11.10}$$

For this experiment the model embodied the Hill equation with the following parameters:

$$y(t) = \frac{v^{2.98}}{(v^{2.98} + 0.404^{2.98})} \tag{11.11}$$

whereas in the actual system the nonlinearity was assumed to be of the following form:

$$y(t) = 0.50 + 0.50 \tanh(6(v(t) - 0.70)) \tag{11.12}$$

The values of $y_0 = 0.5$, $\gamma_0 = 0.50$, $\beta = 6$, and $v_0 = 0.70$ are typical values for this function (see Figure 11.1 for typical shapes of this function).

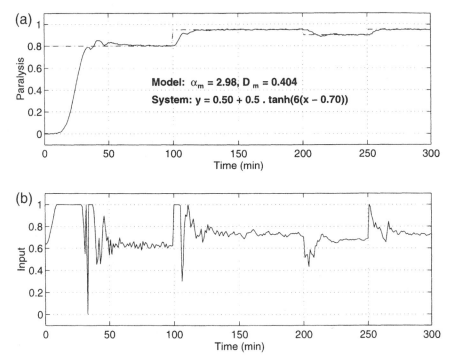

Figure 11.15 Nonlinear GPC with structural nonlinearity mismatch: the model nonlinearity is represented by the Hill equation, whereas the actual system assumed the Meager *et al.* (1989) nonlinearity, $T(z^{-1}) = (1 - 0.8z^{-1})^2$ with additive output noise. (a) Solid line: paralysis; dashdot line: target. (b) Input signal.

With the noise added to the system output, the run produced the output response of Figure 11.15 where despite a slight overshoot, the controller behaved well without deteriorating the quality of the control signal, in spite of the large model mismatch. Another run using the linear GPC algorithm with the actual system assuming the nonlinearity of equation (11.12) produced the output of Figure 11.16 where it can be seen that the performance was inferior to that of Figure 11.15.

11.3.4   Nonlinear GPC in case of large time delays

As pointed out by Agarwal and Seborg (1987), the major benefit of nonlinear controllers can be seen with systems that exhibit large dead-time values. Taking into account this consideration the time delay in equation (11.1) was increased to 4, a noise sequence was superimposed on the output, and the nonlinearity mismatch was considered. The parameter estimates were all 0 except $\hat{b}_1$ (see Section 2.4.1) which was taken to be 1, and the above observer polynomial was also used. The control horizon was taken to be 1. The linear GPC controller led to the performance of Figure 11.17 where it can be seen that the output was too slow to reach higher targets and the input signal too active, especially with high set-points. In contrast, the nonlinear controller's performance of Figure 11.18 was better in terms of input signal and set-point tracking ability of the corresponding output.

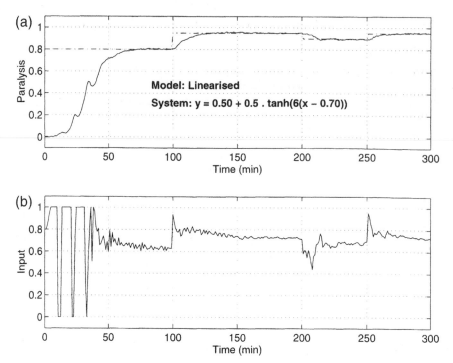

Figure 11.16   Linear GPC of muscle relaxation $NU = 1$, $T(z^{-1}) = (1 - 0.8z^{-1})^2$; the actual system assumed the Meager *et al.* (1989) nonlinearity. (a) Solid line: paralysis; dashdot line: target. (b) Input signal.

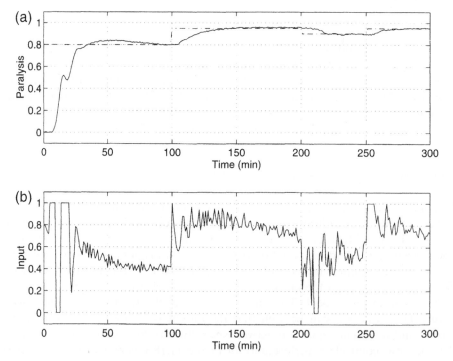

Figure 11.17   Standard linear GPC; $T(z^{-1}) = (1 - 0.8z^{-1})^2$ and noise, delay = 4 min. (a) Solid line: paralysis; dashdot line: target. (b) Input signal.

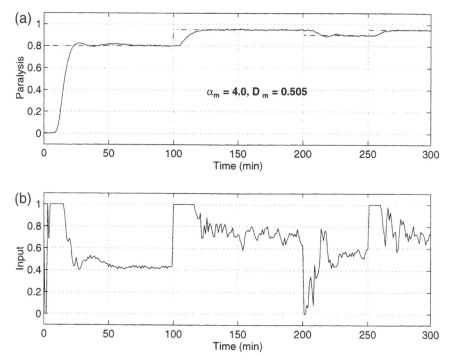

Figure 11.18 Nonlinear GPC; mismatch case, golden section solution $T(z^{-1}) = (1 - 0.8z^{-1})^2$ and noise, delay = 4 min. (a) Solid line: paralysis; dashdot line: target. (b) Input signal.

11.3.5 Nonlinear GPC with bolus doses and pre-specified set-points

This series of simulations dealt with the application of nonlinear GPC using two different patterns of set-points (with anticipated tolerances) for two common types of operations which were provided by an experienced anaesthetist (d'Hollander, 1992) and which were detailed in Chapter 9. The conditions for the experiments were similar to those of the above sections. An initial drug infusion level of 28 was applied for one sample in order to mimic the initial bolus injection normally administered by anaesthetists in the operating theatre.

During that period the loop was open and remained so until the output (paralysis level) reached the safety level of 90% where the loop was closed using GPC with the same initial parameter estimates as in the previous sections. The parameter estimation routine was started three minutes after the loop was closed. The set-point changes were known to the algorithm N_2 samples in advance (anaesthetists know when changes in surgical conditions are likely to happen). The experiments conducted were based on *Pattern A* and *Pattern B* already mentioned in Chapter 9.

A mismatch between the Hill equation parameters in the model and those in the system was considered using the standard deviations mentioned in Section 11.1. A noise sequence similar to that used above was superimposed on the output and therefore a polynomial $T(z^{-1})$ was used to filter the various signals for the controller and estimator. A typical experiment involving *Pattern A* and *Pattern B* produced the outputs of Figures 11.19 and 11.20 where, despite the early reaction of the con-

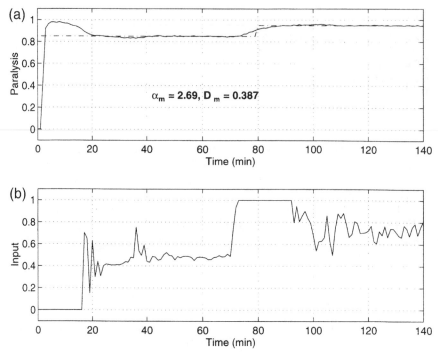

Figure 11.19   Nonlinear GPC; d'Hollander profile, *Pattern A*, bolus dose $T(z^{-1}) = (1 - 0.8z^{-1})^2$ and noise. (a) Solid line: paralysis; dashdot line: target. (b) Input signal.

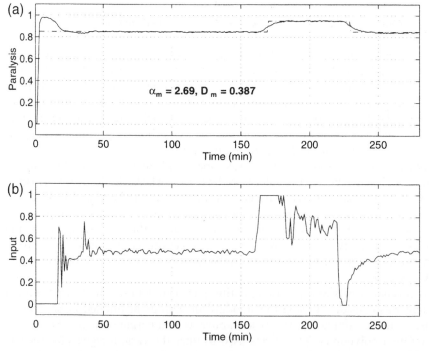

Figure 11.20   Nonlinear GPC; d'Hollander profile, *Pattern B*, bolus dose $T(z^{-1}) = (1 - 0.8z^{-1})^2$ and noise. (a) Solid line: paralysis; dashdot line: target. (b) Input signal.

Table 11.1 Table representing the performance criteria for the standard GPC and the proposed nonlinear controller; * indicates the proposed nonlinear controller.

ISE and ITAE performance criteria		
Figure number	ISE	ITAE
11.3	6.9	649
11.7*	5.9	422
11.4	6.6	440
11.9*	5.9	367
11.5	6.6	495
11.10*	6.6	477
11.6	6.7	606
11.11*	6.3	491
11.16	18	1015
11.15*	13.6	658
11.17	8.9	954
11.18*	9.0	663

troller, the system tracked the new target at the time of change and this with the help of a reasonably active signal.

11.4 Objective comparison between linear GPC and the new nonlinear controller

In order to complement the visual indications of control performance from these experiments, an objective measure of performance over the simulation runs was made using ISE (integral of square errors) and ITAE (integral of time against absolute error) criteria. Table 11.1 gives the ISE and ITAE values for both algorithms in the deterministic and stochastic cases.

As seen in Table 11.1 almost all ISEs and ITAEs obtained with the new controller are lower than the ones which were obtained using the standard GPC algorithm; for instance, the ITAE criteria, which tend to penalise responses for poor set-point tracking, are much lower with the new proposed controller than with the standard GPC algorithm.

11.5 Conclusions

Self-tuning adaptive control techniques have emerged over the past 25 years as a powerful tool for solving highly complex systems that exhibit large varying time delays, varying dynamics, offsets, etc. One of the major hurdles in their development and widespread use is the nonlinearity problem. One method to solve this problem is to assume that the system is linear around the operating point at which it is functioning. Such a strategy has led to many successes, although sometimes at the expense of either robustness or performance, which are themselves in conflict. In simulation as well as in clinical trials we used set-points of 0.8 (20% EMG) and up to 0.85 (15% EMG), although regulation around 0.95 paralysis which are hard to realise with linearised structures, are preferred. In this present study, a nonlinear controller is proposed based on a particular nonlinearity representation which is commonly encountered in biomedicine. It consists of obtaining a linear signal from the nonlinear measured output which is used to estimate the linear model parameters and a cost function which (taking into account the nonlinear prediction) is optimised to obtain a control solution. The golden section search method, the modified simplex method of Nelder–Mead and genetic algorithms have been used for this purpose. A comparison with the linear GPC controller has shown that the scheme leads to better results in the region close to saturation (difficult area of the nonlinear static function) in both deterministic and stochastic cases, even when a large time delay and large mismatch (well beyond the reported standard deviation values) between the assumed model nonlinearity and the true system nonlinearity are considered; this is clinically important since surgeons often require a 0.9 level of relaxation for light surgery followed by a 0.95 level when deep incisions are made. Furthermore, it has been shown that even when the wrong nonlinearity structure was assumed the controller proved robust without increasing the control signal activity. It is also worth noting that the proposed scheme allows one to retain the advantages of the observer and model-following polynomial design features which have been demonstrated to improve the controller's performance and give it more flexibility.

CHAPTER TWELVE

Conclusions and Further Work

12.1 Summary of the book's main contributions

There is no doubt that the underlying message which stems from the work described in this book is that generalised predictive control (GPC) has proven, as it has done in other areas, to be a powerful control tool in biomedicine and particularly in anaesthesia, able to solve complex problems and achieve tight objectives without compromising on performance. Hence, the main contributions of this work can be summarised as follows.

- We have described the development of a feedback control system for atracurium drug delivery based on a single-input single-output (SISO) version of GPC. After extensive simulation experiments, the closed-loop system was successfully applied to patients in theatre at two sites (Glasgow Western Infirmary and Sheffield Royal Hallamshire Hospital) during surgical procedures which required muscle relaxation. During these trials excellent regulation with minimum drug consumption was achieved. Moreover, of the many features characterising the system, we can cite that:

  (a) It is easy to use by the medical practitioners as it requires only basic knowledge of computers.

  (b) The small size of the software is easily transferable to any IBM compatible machine with minimum memory capacity, and because of the relatively long sampling time used (1 minute) processor speed does not represent a major requirement.

  (c) The SISO GPC algorithm, with filtering capabilities of the observer polynomial $T(z^{-1})$, has proved robust over a wide range of patients' dynamics (in terms of dynamical variations, disturbance rejection and uncertainties (unmodelled dynamics)), and also against diathermy (electrical interference). It is flexible; the easy understanding of its tuning 'knobs' meant that various response characteristics could be obtained for various surgical conditions.

  (d) Built-in procedures check the integrity of data exchange between the computer, the Relaxograph measuring device and the syringe pump unit and alert the user of any violation, making therefore the whole control system safe to use.

- We have shown that the use of SISO GPC in a fixed mode (patient's model not updated) with a measurement variable is more advantageous (in terms of model mismatch) than the use of a target concentration infusion (TCI) system which is an open-loop configuration for controlling anaesthesia. The fixed GPC uses mean arterial pressure (MAP) as an inferential variable which is considered to be a good indicator for unconsciousness.

- The extension of the SISO work to the multivariable case in which simultaneous control and on-line identification of muscle relaxation via EMG measurements and unconsciousness via MAP measurements has been described. A multivariable model for anaesthesia was derived upon which the multivariable study was based. A control system based on the multivariable version of GPC was not an easy task to accomplish due to the various problems associated with communicating with four devices at the same time (two measuring devices and two actuators), each having its own protocol. The resultant system produced was applied in theatre (at Glasgow Western Infirmary) during three surgical procedures, one of them being the revolutionary keyhole operation. Success in terms of maintaining reasonable muscle paralysis levels as well as reasonable bounds on systolic arterial pressure (SAP) was obtained. Further, improvements are being made to the system in terms of communication protocols, it being hoped to conduct more clinical trials in the future.

- Because GPC's control sequence stems from the optimisation of a well-defined cost function, we reckon that the work would be incomplete without tackling the issue of constraints. In anaesthesia therapy, these constraints are well defined since the anaesthetist knows the minimum and maximum bounds of the various variables involved for each type of surgery. In order to include the constraints within the optimisation function, the quadratic programming approach (QP), as described by Lawson and Hanson (1974), was invoked. Although this method is computationally expensive, it is known for its good stability properties and for allowing the inclusion of all types of constraints, e.g. input magnitude, input rate, and output constraints. Significant improvements over the standard GPC algorithm were obtained with a well-behaved output together with better control signal activity. Perhaps the issue which dominated the various experiments was that of constraints' incompatibility where a solution to the problem could not be found taking into account all the constraints. This reflects the nature of most engineering problems where it is not always possible to solve them uniquely. Hence, a method was proposed and studied in which the constraints causing incompatibility were removed until a solution was found.

- We have given due attention to the issue of model representation and estimation. First, given the structure of the multivariable anaesthesia model, i.e. a two-input two-output system with only one interaction path, it seemed more logical to see it as two single independent loops with the one-way interaction represented as a feedforward path. This had the advantage of reducing the computational burden, and also reducing the levels of interactions. Second, and in a separate study, instead of the patient's model being updated using the standard recursive least-squares estimation scheme (RLS), the long range control predictions were included in an estimation scheme, named long range predictive identification (LRPI), which goes beyond the one-step ahead prediction idea and includes the same horizon as that of the control sequence. Although this was found to increase the control signals' activity for control horizons of $NU > 1$, the disturbance rejection properties were better than in the standard RLS case.

- Nowadays, the issue of intelligent control systems (based on artificial intelligence) dominates many scientific gatherings, and in an attempt to face up to the challenge offered by these systems, a section is included where multivariable GPC is compared to multivariable self-organising fuzzy logic control (SOFLC) (which is classified as an intelligent approach) using the multivariable anaesthesia model as a test bed. The results obtained were not surprising (predictable!) in that they reflected the characteristics of both controllers' categories (a model-based approach and an intelligent approach), i.e. when the system's mathematical model is known and is structurally accurate then multivariable GPC proves to be more robust than SOFLC. It is worth noting that care should be exercised when claiming that fuzzy logic control does not use a process model since the process knowledge is also embedded in the fuzzy logic structure except that it is linguistic rather than analytical.

- We can capitalise on the power of GPC to include knowledge about the set-points directly into the control sequence calculation. In anaesthesia, such knowledge is available and hence can be incorporated in the algorithm for optimal performance. This performance has been assessed from two aspects: first, in the SISO case, the algorithm converges to the new specified target quicker and in the multi-input multi-output (MIMO) case, full decoupling in the low and mid-frequency range can be achieved. Hence, using nominal surgical set-point profiles provided to us by an experienced anaesthetist, SISO GPC was able to fulfil the predefined constraints while producing good overall performances, and in the MIMO case the levels of interactions from the blood pressure channel in the muscle relaxation channel were kept at their minimum, making the concept of pre-specified (or pre-programmed) set-points an attractive and elegant scheme.

- GPC's versatility was tested when an autonomous structure was given to the multivariable adaptive controller by adding a hierarchical supervisory level in the form of a fault detection isolation accommodation scheme (FDIA). Although various alarms are normally fitted to all equipment used in the operating theatre, the FDIA algorithm superimposed on the GPC procedure allows the controller to branch to other tasks without the need for interrupting its operation. The nature of the new task to which GPC branches is determined by the nature of the fault detected (diagnosis and operation). Although not yet tested in the operating theatre, the augmented algorithm performed well in simulations by detecting, diagnosing and accommodating for the various faults normally encountered under operating conditions.

- Finally, we have shown that GPC can be configured to absorb the system's nonlinearity not only by linearising the process around an operating point but also by including the nonlinear predictions in the optimisation process in a scheme named nonlinear generalised predictive control (NLGPC) and this seems to produce better results even when a relatively large mismatch exists between the model considered and the actual system. In the simulation study that we conducted, and in order to obtain the control sequence, we experimented with various optimisation techniques including genetic algorithms which have the advantages of:

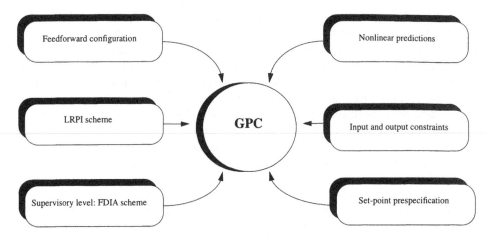

Figure 12.1   The various schemes added to GPC to give it a universal structure.

(a) Not requiring a gradient of the function being optimised.
(b) Avoiding local extrema.

- It is evident from the above contributions that this work has placed emphasis on a gradual build-up of a kind of a jigsaw puzzle starting from a simple and yet ingenious algorithm which is GPC and arriving at a configuration which includes all the necessary accessories which allow for optimal results as shown in Figure 12.1. Long before that, GPC alone was known as the 'universal controller'. The configuration of Figure 12.1, however, could be called the 'complete controller'.

12.2   Future work

There is no doubt that research in control has been dominated recently by intelligent themes such as neural networks, fuzzy logic, and genetic algorithms. As a result, various synergies have been described between fuzzy logic and neural networks (the concept of neuro-fuzzy control) (Nie and Linkens, 1995), and fuzzy logic and genetic algorithms (Linkens and Nyongesa, 1995) which not only showed that these intelligent structures can interact together but also can make the overall structure more robust against uncertainties as well as disturbances.

We hope that through the study that we conducted in Chapter 8 in which GPC was compared with SOFLC we have reinforced the idea that when a good model of a process exists then a model-based approach is recommended, but if uncertainties are suspected or variables cannot be accessed, then an intelligent control structure should be found more advantageous. Therefore, we belong to the category of researchers who would rather reconcile than confront, as far as the issue of robustness is concerned. This is very much part of the future work we intend to pursue, particularly that of establishing synergisms between mathematical model-based approaches and intelligent approaches. An example of this is the synergy between

GPC and SOFLC where the former can be used as a mechanism to make the latter adjust itself to improve the system's performance. The configuration is shown in Figure 12.2 and the resulting controller is called a predictive self-organising fuzzy logic controller (PSOFLC).

The idea behind the new algorithm is to replace the performance index table (see Chapter 8) in the fuzzy logic controller with a different mechanism that will allow the rules modifier to create, delete and alter rules in the same way in which a self-organising fuzzy logic control scheme normally behaves. Since the index used for the rules modifier algorithm is an incremental quantity which excites the rule generation process, we propose to replace it with the increment generated by GPC whose parameters are adjusted by a parameter estimation algorithm, namely RLS. Hence, with this scheme equation (8.2) becomes:

$$E(nT - mT) \rightarrow CE(nT - mT) \rightarrow U(nT - mT) + G_{\delta u_1} \delta u_1(nT) \qquad (12.1)$$

where $\delta u_1(nT)$ is the increment generated by GPC, and this will represent the basis upon which the adaptation is carried out.

A series of simulations have been conducted using both the new proposed scheme of PSOFLC and SOFLC and their performances were compared using the muscle relaxation process as a test bed. Figures 12.3 and 12.4 show the performances of PSOFLC and SOFLC respectively where it can be seen that the performance achieved with the new integrated scheme was better.

We strongly believe that other interesting synergies between these intelligent systems exist and that this is only one of them. Further research in this particular direction deserves serious consideration because we feel that between model-based approaches and intelligent approaches there should certainly be rapprochement rather than conflict.

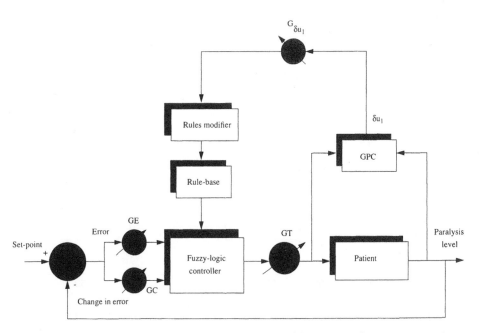

Figure 12.2   Schematic diagram representing the structure of the PSOFLC idea.

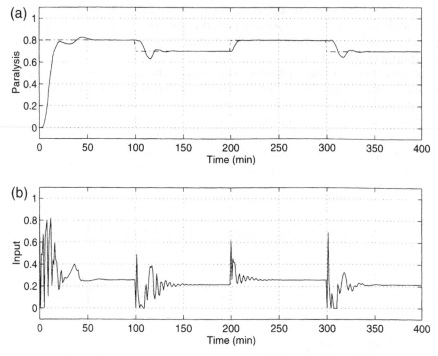

Figure 12.3   SOFLC of the muscle relaxation process. (a) Solid line: paralysis; dashdot line: target. (b) Input signal.

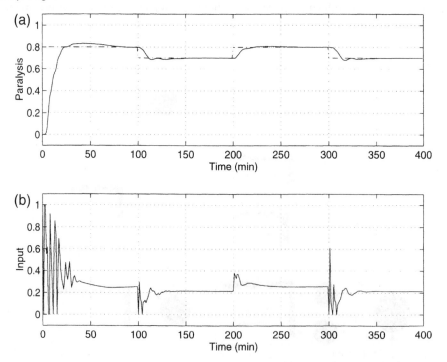

Figure 12.4   PSOFLC of the muscle relaxation process. (a) Solid line: paralysis; dashdot line: target. (b) Input signal.

Modelling of Multivariable System Dynamics

Modelling of multivariable system dynamics is usually expressed in terms of a set of ordinary differential equations which can be translated into the state-space form:

$$\begin{cases} \dot{x}(t) = Ax(t) + Bu(t - \tau_{ij}) \\ y(t) = Cx(t) + Du(t) \end{cases} \tag{I.1}$$

where $x(t)$, $u(t)$ and $y(t)$ are $(n \times 1)$, $(r \times 1)$ and $(m \times 1)$ vectors representing the state, the input and the output variables respectively. A, B, C and D are matrices characterizing the system dynamics, and τ_{ij} the pure time delay for the ijth element of B.

The Laplace transform of the above system is given by:

$$\begin{cases} sX(s) - x(0) = AX(s) + e^{-\tau_{ij}s}BU(s) \\ Y(s) = CX(s) + DU(s) \end{cases} \tag{I.2}$$

Assuming zero initial conditions and rearranging to solve for $X(s)$ yields:

$$\begin{cases} Y(s) = G(s)U(s) \\ G(s) = C[SI_n - A]^{-1}B\,e^{-\tau_{ij}s} + D \end{cases} \tag{I.3}$$

The continuous-time state-space equations of system (I.2) have an equivalent time representation which is generally given by:

$$\begin{cases} x[(t + 1)h] = \Phi x(ht) + \Delta u[(t - k_{ij})h] \\ y(ht) = Hx(ht) + Lu(ht) \end{cases} \tag{I.4}$$

where h is the sampling time and t is the time index $t = 0, 1, 2, \ldots$. The matrices Φ and Δ can be evaluated using discrete integration of the continuous-time equations expressed in system (I.2) or using Laplace transforms. Using the z operator on system equations (I.4) and dropping h for simplicity's sake leads to:

$$\begin{cases} x(t) = [zI_n - \Phi]^{-1}z^{k_{ij}}u(t) \\ y(t) = Hx(t) + Lu(t) \end{cases} \tag{I.5}$$

Substituting one equation into another in the above system results in the following equation:

$$\begin{cases} y(t) = G(z^{-1})u(t) \\ G(z^{-1}) = H[zI_n - \Phi]^{-1}\Delta z^{-k_{ij}} + L \end{cases} \tag{I.6}$$

Equation (I.6) is the sampled-data system equivalent to the Laplace transforms relation equation (I.3). Therefore the polynomial transfer function matrix $G(z^{-1})$ can be derived directly from $G(s)$.

For each element $G(s)$, the corresponding function of z is given by:

$$G_{ij}(z^{-1}) = Z\left\{\frac{(1 - e^{-sh})G_{ij}(s)}{s}\right\} \tag{I.7}$$

where

$$\frac{1 - e^{-sh}}{s}$$

is the transfer function of the zero-order hold which is most commonly used as data extrapolator. The polynomial transfer function matrix can be written as:

$$G(z^{-1}) = \begin{bmatrix} \dfrac{G_{n_{11}}}{G_{d_{11}}} & \cdots & \dfrac{G_{n_{1r}}}{G_{d_{1r}}} \\ \vdots & \cdots & \vdots \\ \dfrac{G_{n_{m1}}}{G_{d_{m1}}} & \cdots & \dfrac{G_{n_{mr}}}{G_{d_{mr}}} \end{bmatrix} \tag{I.8}$$

Reducing these polynomial fractions into their common denominator row by row leads to the following:

$$G'_{n_{ij}}(z^{-1}) = G_{n_{ij}} \times \prod_{\substack{k=1 \\ k \neq j}}^{r} G_{d_{ik}}(z^{-1}) \quad \text{for } i = 1, \ldots, m$$

$$G'_{d_{ii}}(z^{-1}) = \prod_{k=1}^{m} G_{d_{ik}}(z^{-1}) \quad \text{for } k = 1, \ldots, m$$

Using these equations, the transfer function matrix $G(z^{-1})$ can be written in terms of $Gn(z^{-1})$ and $Gd(z^{-1})$ as:

$$G_n(z^{-1}) = \begin{bmatrix} G'_{n_{11}} & \cdots & G'_{n_{1r}} \\ \vdots & \cdots & \vdots \\ G'_{n_{m1}} & \cdots & G'_{n_{mr}} \end{bmatrix} \quad \text{and} \quad G_d(z^{-1}) = \begin{bmatrix} \dfrac{1}{G'_{d_{11}}} & 0 & 0 & 0 \\ 0 & \dfrac{1}{G'_{d_{22}}} & & \cdots \\ \vdots & \vdots & \vdots & \cdots \\ 0 & 0 & 0 & \dfrac{1}{G'_{d_{mm}}} \end{bmatrix}$$

Consider now partitioning the input vector $uz(t)$ into $(mx\ 1)$ vector $u(t)$, and $(mx\ 1)$ vector $\xi(t)$ of random variables, such that:

$$G_n(z^{-1}) = [z^{-k_{ij}}B(z^{-1})C(z^{-1})]\begin{bmatrix} u(t) \\ \Phi(t) \end{bmatrix}$$

and $A(z^{-1}) = Gd(z^{-1})$.

Therefore system equations (I.6) can be written as:

$$A(z^{-1})y(t) = z^{-k_{ij}}B(z^{-1})u(t) + C(z^{-1})\xi(t) \tag{I.9}$$

or including the Δ operator, equation (I.9) becomes:

$$A(z^{-1})\Delta y(t) = z^{-k_{ij}}B(z^{-1})\Delta u(t) + C(z^{-1})\xi(t) \tag{I.10}$$

$A(z^{-1})$ and $C(z^{-1})$ are diagonal matrices as it has been established. Details on the estimation routine are given in Appendix II.

Finally, as pointed out earlier, this representation is typical of many industrial processes, although additional interactions between different outputs could in fact be a possibility.

Recursive Least-squares Algorithm: the Multivariable Case

$$y_t^i = x_t^{i^T}\hat{\theta}_t^i + \varepsilon_t^i \quad \text{for } i = 1, 2, \ldots, p \tag{II.1}$$

where

y_t^i is the ith component of the output vector y_t
ε_t^i is the ith component of the residual vector ε_t
x_t^i is the data vector
θ_t^i is the associated parameter vector

From the standard recursive least-squares algorithm, the parameters are found using the following algorithm assuming that the A_i matrices are diagonal:

$$\hat{\theta}_{t+1}^i = \hat{\theta}_t^i + \gamma_t p_{t+1} x_{t+1} [y_{t+1}^i - x^T \theta_i^i] \tag{II.2}$$

where

$$x_t^i = [y_{t-1}^i, y_{t-2}^i, \ldots, y_{t-na}^i, u_{t-1}^1, \ldots, u_{t-nb}^1, \ldots, u_{t-1}^p, \ldots, u_{t-nb}^p]^T$$

Since the measurement vectors are different for every channel, the gain γ and the covariance matrix p_t need to be updated p times in addition to the updating of the parameters $\hat{\theta}_i$.

Recursive Least-squares Algorithm: the Multivariable Case

Converting the LSI Problem to the LDP Problem: the Constrained Solution

Let k denote the rank of the $m_2 \times n$ matrix A in LSI problem (5.1). In order to convert the LSI problem to an LDP problem an orthogonal decomposition of the matrix A is necessary. Either a QR or a singular value decomposition value (SVD)

$$A = Q \begin{bmatrix} R & 0 \\ 0 & 0 \end{bmatrix} K^{\mathrm{T}} \equiv [Q_1 : Q_2] \begin{bmatrix} R & 0 \\ 0 & 0 \end{bmatrix} \begin{bmatrix} K_1^{\mathrm{T}} \\ K_2^{\mathrm{T}} \end{bmatrix} \tag{III.1}$$

where Q is ($m_2 \times m_2$) orthogonal, K is ($n \times n$) orthogonal and R is ($k \times k$) orthogonal.

Let us introduce the orthogonal change of variables:

$$x = K_1 y \tag{III.2}$$

The objective function to be minimised in the LSI problem can then be written as:

$$\phi(x) = \| Ax - b \|^2 = \left\| \begin{bmatrix} Ry \\ 0 \end{bmatrix} - \begin{bmatrix} Q_1^{\mathrm{T}}b \\ Q_2^{\mathrm{T}}b \end{bmatrix} \right\|^2 = \| Ry - \tilde{b}_1 \|^2 + \| \tilde{b}_2 \|^2 \tag{III.3}$$

where

$$\tilde{b}_i = Q_i^{\mathrm{T}}b \quad \text{for } i = 1, 2 \tag{III.4}$$

With a further change of variables:

$$z = Ry - \tilde{b}_1 \tag{III.5}$$

we may write:

$$\phi(x) = \| z \|^2 + \| \tilde{b}_2 \|^2 \tag{III.6}$$

The original LSI problem of minimising $\| Ax - b \|$ subject to $Cx \geq h$ is thus equivalent to the following LDP problem, except for the additive constant $\| \tilde{b}_2 \|$ in the objective function:

Minimise $\| z \|$

subject to: $CK_1 R^{-1} \geq h - CK_1 R^{-1} \tilde{b}_1$

(III.7)

If a vector $\hat{z}$ is computed as a solution of this LDP problem, then a solution vector $\hat{x}$ for the original LSI problem can be computed from equations (III.5) and (III.2). The squared residual vector norm for the original problem can be computed from equation (III.6).

References

AGARWAL, M. and SEBORG, D. E., 1987, Self-tuning controllers for nonlinear systems, *Automatica*, **23**, 2, 209–214.

AL-ASSAF, Y., 1988, 'Self-tuning control: theory and applications', unpublished DPhil. thesis, Oxford University, Oxford, UK.

ALVIS, J. M., REVES, J. G., SPAIN, J. A. and SHEPPARD, L. C., 1985, Computer-assisted continuous infusion of the intravenous analgesic fentanyl during general anaesthesia – an interactive system, *Institution of Electrical and Electronic Engineers Transactions on Biomedical Engineering*, **BME-32**, 323–329.

ASBURY, A. J., 1990, unpublished correspondence letter.

ASBURY, A. J., BROWN, B. H. and LINKENS, D. A., 1980, Control of neuromuscular blockade by external feedback mechanism, *British Journal of Anaesthesia*, **52**, 633p–634p.

ASSILIAN, S. and MAMDANI, E. H., 1974, An experiment in linguistic synthesis with a fuzzy logic controller, *International Journal of Man–Machine Studies*, **7**, 1–13.

ASTROM, K. J., 1992, Autonomous controllers, Proceedings of the IFAC Conference on Artificial Intelligence in Real-time Control, Delft, Holland, June, 1–6.

ASTROM, K. J. and WITTENMARK, B., 1973, On self-tuning regulators, *Automatica*, **9**, 185.

ASTROM, K. J. and WITTENMARK, B., 1984, *Computer-controlled Systems–Theory and Design*, Prentice-Hall, Inc., Englewood Cliffs, New Jersey, USA.

ASTROM, K. J. and WITTENMARK, B., 1989, *Adaptive Control*, Addison-Wesley, Reading, Mass., USA.

BARS, R. and HABER, R., 1988, Long-range predictive control of nonlinear systems given by volterra series, *Preprints of the Symposium on Identification and System Parameter Estimation*, **2**, 931–935.

BARS, R. and HABER, R., 1991, Weighted one-step ahead adaptive predictive control of nonlinear processes, *Preprints of the IMACS Symposium*, Lille, France, 16–21.

BELANGER, P. R., 1983, On type-I systems and the Clarke-Gawthrop regulator, *Automatica*, **19**, 91–94.

BELLMAN, R., 1971, Topics in pharmacokinetics III: Repeated dosage and impulse control, *Mathematical Biosciences*, **12**, 1–5.

BENEKEN, J. E. W. and GRAVENSTEIN, J. S., 1987, Sophisticated alarms in patient monitoring: A methodology based on systems engineering concepts, in Ravenstein, J. S., Newbower, R. S., Ream, A. K. and Smith, N. T. (Eds) *The Automated Anaesthesia Record and Alarm Systems*, Butterworths, Boston, USA, 211–228.

BIERMAN, G. J., 1977, *Factorization Methods for Discrete Sequential Estimation*, Academic Press, New York, USA.

BIRKS, R., HUXLEY, H. E. and KATZ, B., 1960, The fine structure of neuromuscular junction, *Journal of Physiology (London)*, **150**, 134.

BITMEAD, R. R., GEVERS, M. and WERTZ, V., 1990, *Adaptive Optimal Control – the Thinking Man's GPC*, Prentice-Hall, New York, USA.

BLOM, J. A., DE RUYTER, J. A. F., SARANUMMI, N. and BENEKEN, J. E. W., 1985, Detection of trends in monitored variables, in Carson, E. R. and Cramp, D. G. (Eds) *Computers and Control in Clinical Medicine*, Plenum Press, New York, USA, 153–174.

BLUELL, J., JELLIFE, R., KALABA, R. and SRIDHAR, R., 1969, Modern control theory and optimal drug regimes, *Mathematical Biosciences*, **5**, 285–296.

BOHM, J., HALOUSKOVA, A., KARNY, M. and PETERKA, V., 1984, Simple LQ self-tuning regulators, 9th IFAC World Congress, Budapest, Hungary.

BORTOLOTTO, G. and JØRGENSEN, S. B., 1986, Finite horizon multivariable optimal control of constrained chemical processes. IFAC 6th World Congress, London, UK.

BRADLOW, H. S. and O'MAHONY, J. R., 1990, PC-based muscle relaxation controller and monitor, Annual Conference of the Institution of Electrical and Electronic Engineers Engineering in Medicine and Biology Society, 947–948.

BRECKENRIDGE, J. L. and AITKENHEAD, A. R., 1983, Awareness during anaesthesia: a review, *Annals of the Royal College of Surgeons of England*, **6**, 93–96.

BROWN, B. H., ASBURY, A. J., LINKENS, D. A., PERKS, P. and ANTHONY, M., 1980, Closed-loop control of muscle relaxation during surgery, *Clinical Physics and Physiological Measurement*, **1**, 203–210.

CASS, N. M., LAMPARD, D. G., BROWN, W. A. and COLES, J. R., 1976, Computer-controlled muscle relaxation: a comparison of four muscle relaxants in sheep, *Anaesthesia in Intensive Care*, **4**, 16–22.

CHILCOAT, R. T., 1980, A review of the control of depth of anaesthesia, *Transactions of the Institute of Measurement and Control*, **2**, 38–45.

CLARKE, D. W., 1985, Implementation of self-tuning controllers, in Harris, C. J. and Billings, S. A. (Eds) *Self-tuning and Adaptive Control: Theory and Application*, Institution of Electrical Engineers Control Engineering, **15**, 146–147.

CLARKE, D. W., 1994, *Advances in Model-based Predictive Control*, Oxford University Press, Oxford, UK.

CLARKE, D. W. and GAWTHROP, P. J., 1975, Self-tuning controller, *Institution of Electrical Engineers Proceedings, Pt D, Control Theory and Applications*, **122**, 9, 929–934.

CLARKE, D. W. and GAWTHROP, P. J., 1979, Self-tuning control, *Institution of Electrical Engineers Proceedings, Pt D, Control Theory and Applications*, **126**, 633–640.

CLARKE, D. W. and SCATTOLINI, R., 1991, Constrained receding-horizon predictive control, *Institution of Electrical Engineers Proceedings, Pt D, Control Theory and Applications*, **138**, 347–354.

CLARKE, D. W., MOHTADI, C. and TUFFS, P. S., 1987a, Generalised predictive control – part I. The basic algorithm, *Automatica*, **23**, 2, 137–148.

CLARKE, D. W., MOHTADI, C. and TUFFS, P. S., 1987b, Generalised predictive control – part II. Extensions and interpretations, *Automatica*, **23**, 2, 149–160.

CUTLER, C. R. and RAMAKER, B. L., 1980, Dynamic matrix control – A computer control algorithm, Paper WP5-B, Proceedings of the Joint Automatic Control Conference, San Francisco, USA.

DALE, H. H. and FELDBERG, W., 1934, Chemical transmission at motor nerve endings in voluntary muscle, *Journal of Physiology (London)*, **81**, 39.

DALEY, S. and GILL, K. F., 1986, A design study of a self-organising fuzzy logic controller, *Proceedings of the Institution of Mechanical Engineers*, **200**, 59–69.

DE KEYSER, R. M. C. and VAN CAUWENBERGHE, A. R., 1979a, A self-tuning predictor as operator guide, 5th IFAC Symposium on Identification and System Parameter Estimation, Darmstadt, Germany.

DE KEYSER, R. M. C. and VAN CAUWENBERGHE, A. R., 1979b, A self-tuning multistep predictor application, *Automatica*, **17**, 167–174.

DE KEYSER, R. M. C. and VAN CAUWENBERGHE, A. R., 1983, Microcomputer-controlled servo system based on self-tuning adaptive long-range prediction, in Tsafestas, S. G. and Hamza, M. H. (Eds) *Methods and Applications of Measurement and Control*, 583–587.

DE KEYSER, R. M. C. and VAN CAUWENBERGHE, A. R., 1985, Extended prediction self-adaptive control, 7th IFAC Symposium on Identification and System Parameter Estimation, Invited Session on Applications of Adaptive and Self-tuning Control, York, UK, 1255–1260.

DENAI, M., LINKENS, D. A., ASBURY, A. J., MACLEOD, A. D. and GRAY, M. W., 1990, Self-tuning PID control of Atracurium-induced muscle relaxation in surgical patients, *Institution of Electrical Engineers Proceedings, Pt D, Control Theory and Applications*, **137**, 261–272.

D'HOLLANDER, A., 1992, Private communication.

EBERT, J., CARROL, S. K. and BRADLEY, E. L., 1986, Closed-loop feedback control of muscle relaxation with vecuronium in surgical patients, *Anaesthesia and Anesthesiology*, **65**, S44.

FAVIER, G., 1987, Self-tuning long-range predictive controllers, Proceedings of the IFAC World Congress, Munich, Germany.

FLETCHER, R., 1980, *Practical Methods of Optimisation*, John Wiley & Sons Ltd, Chichester, UK.

GARCIA, G. E., 1984, Quadratic dynamic matrix control of nonlinear processes, Proceedings of the Annual AIChE Meeting, San Francisco, USA, F3–G13.

GARCIA, G. E. and MORSHEDI, A. M., 1986, Quadratic programming solution of dynamic matrix control (QDMC), *Chemical Engineering Communications*, **46**, 73–87.

GAWTHROP, P. J., 1977, Some interpretations of the self-tuning controller, *Institution of Electrical Engineers Proceedings, Pt D, Control Theory and Applications*, **124**, 10, 889–894.

GENTRY, W. B., KREJCIE, T. C., HENTHORN, T. K., SHANKS, C. A., GUPTA, D. K. and AVRAM, M. J., 1993, Infusion rate-related thiopental dose response: application of a kinetic-dynamic model, *Anesthesiology*, **79**, A339.

GEPTS, E., CAMU, F., COCKSHOTT, I. D. and DOUGLAS, E. J., 1987, Disposition of propofol administered as constant rate intravenous infusions in humans, *Anaesthesia and Analgesia*, **66**, 1256–1263.

GEPTS, E., JONCKHEER, K., MAES, V., SONCK, W. and CAMU, F., 1988, Disposition kinetics of propofol during alfentanil anaesthesia, *Anaesthesia (Supplement)*, **43**, 8–13.

GOLDBERG, E., 1989, *Genetic Algorithms in Search, Optimisation, and Machine Learning*, Addison-Wesley, Reading, Massachusetts, USA.

GOODWIN, G. C. and SIN, K. S., 1984, *Adaptive Filtering Prediction and Control*, Prentice-Hall, Inc., Englewood Cliffs, New Jersey, USA.

GRAUPE, D., 1976, *Identification of Systems*, Robert Krieger Publishing Company, Malabar, Florida, USA.

GRAY, W. M. and ASBURY, A. J., 1986, Measurement and control of depth of anaesthesia in surgical patients, 3rd IMEKO Conference on Measurement in Clinical Medicine, Edinburgh, UK, 167–172.

GREGORY, P. C., 1959, Proceedings of Self-adaptive Flight Control Symposium, WADC Report.

HALFORD, N. H. G. and SHEINER, L. B., 1981, Understanding the dose–effect relationship: clinical application of pharmacokinetic–pharmacodynamic models, *Clinical Pharmacokinetics*, **6**, 429–453.

HARRIS, C. J. and MOORE, C. G., 1989, 'Intelligent identification and control for autonomous guided vehicles using adaptive fuzzy based algorithms', internal report, Southampton University, Southampton, UK.

HARRIS, C. J. and MOORE, C. G., 1990, Real-time fuzzy-based self-learning predictors and controllers, in *Proceedings of the 11th IFAC World Congress*, Tallinn, USSR, **7**, 180–186.

HEINONEN, P. and NEUVO, Y., 1987, FIT-Median hybrid filters, *Transactions of the Institution of Electrical and Electronic Engineers on Acoustics, Speech, Signal Processing*, **35**, 832–838.

HOLLAND, J. H., 1973, Genetic algorithms and the optimal allocation of trials, *SIAM Journal of Computing*, **2**, No. 2, 89–104.

HOLLAND, J. H., 1975, *Adaptation in Natural and Artificial Systems*, Addison-Wesley, Reading, Massachusetts.

ISERMANN, R., 1981, Fault detection methods for the supervision of technical processes, *Process Automation*, **1**, 36–44.

ISERMANN, R., 1984, Process fault detection based on modeling and estimation methods – A survey, *Automatica*, **20**, 4, 387–404.

ISERMANN, R. and FREYERMUTH, B., 1991, Process fault diagnosis based on process model knowledge. Part I: Principles for fault diagnosis with parameter estimation, *American Society for Mechanical Engineers Journal of Dynamic Systems Measurement and Control*, **113**, 4, 620–626.

JACOBS, J. R., SHAFER, S. L., LARSEN, J. L. and HAWKINS, E. D., 1990, Two equally valid interpretations of the linear multicompartment mammillary pharmacokinetic model, *Journal of Pharmaceutical Sciences*, **79**, 331–333.

JACOBS, J. R. and WILLIAMS, E. A., 1993, Algorithm to control effect compartment drug concentrations in pharmacokinetic model-driven drug delivery, *Institute of Electrical and Electronic Engineers Transactions on Biomedical Engineering*, **40**, 10, 993–999.

JACOBS, O. L. R., BULLINGHAM, R. E. S., McQUAY, H. J. and REASBECK, M. P., 1982, On-line estimation in the control of post-operative pain, Proceedings of the 6th IFAC Symposium on Identification of Systems and Parameter Estimation, Washington, USA.

JANNETT, T. C., 1986, Correspondence letter, *Institution of Electrical and Electronic Engineers Transactions on Biomedical Engineering*, **BME-33**, 722–723.

JANNETT, T. C. and DE FALQUE, R. J., 1990, Integrated instrumentation of closed-loop feedback control of muscle relaxation: Initial clinical trials, Annual Conference of the Institution of Electrical and Electronic Engineers Engineering in Medicine and Biology Society, 945–946.

JEZEK, J. and KUCERA, V., 1986, Efficient algorithm for matrix spectral factorisation, *Automatica*, **21**, 6, 663–669.

KALMAN, R. E., 1958, Design of a self-optimising control system, *American Society of Mechanical Engineers Transactions of Basic Engineering*, **80**, 468–478.

KAM, W. Y., THAM, M. T., MORRIS, A. J. and WARWICK, K., 1985, Multivariable self-tuning: structure identification and control, Proceedings of the IFAC Conference on Identification and Parameter Estimation, York, UK, 385–390.

KING, P. J. and MAMDANI, E. H., 1977, Application of fuzzy control systems to industrial processes, *Automatica*, **13**, 235–242.

KIRKPATRICK, T., COCKSHOTT, I. D., DOUGLAS, E. J. and NIMMO, W. S., 1988, Pharmacokinetics of propofol (Diprivan) in elderly patients, *British Journal of Anaesthesia*, **60**, 146–150.

KOIVO, A. J., 1980, Automatic continuous-time blood pressure control in dogs by means of hypotensive drug injection, *Institute of Electrical and Electronic Engineers Transactions on Biomedical Engineering*, **27**, 574–581.

KOIVO, A. J., 1981, Microprocessor-based controller for pharmacodynamic applications, *Institute of Electrical and Electronic Engineers Transactions on Automatic Control*, **26**, 1208–1213.

KORTMANN, M. and UNBEHAUEN, H., 1987, Identification methods for nonlinear MISO systems, Proceedings of the IFAC World Congress, Munich, Germany, 225–230.

KUCERA, V. and VOSTRY, Z., 1976, Expanding spectral density into a correlation sequence, *Transactions of the Institution of Electrical and Electronic Engineers on Automatic Control*, **21**, 592–593.

KWOK, K. Y., MUTHA, R. K., SHAH, S. L., CLANACHAN, A. S. and FINEGAN, B. A., 1991, Constrained long-range adaptive predictive control of arterial pressure, *International Journal of Adaptive Control and Signal Processing*, **5**, 363–374.

KWOK, K. E., SHAH, S. L., CLANACHAN, A. S. and FINEGAN, B. A., 1995, Evaluation of long-range adaptive predictive controller for computerised drug-delivery systems, *Institute of Electrical and Electronic Engineers Transactions on Biomedical Engineering*, **42**, 79–86.

LAMBERT, M., 1987a, 'Adaptive control of flexible systems', unpublished DPhil. thesis, Oxford University, Oxford, UK.

LAMBERT, E., 1987b, 'The industrial application of long-range prediction', unpublished DPhil. thesis, Oxford University, Oxford, UK.

LAWSON, C. L. and HANSON, R. J., 1974, *Solving Least-Squares Problems*, Prentice-Hall Series in Automatic Computation. Prentice-Hall, Inc., Englewood Cliffs, New Jersey, USA.

LEE, T. H., LIM, K. W. and LAI, W. C., 1991, Real-time multivariable self-tuning controller using a feedforward paradigm with application to a coupled electric-drive pilot plant, *Transactions of the Institution of Electrical and Electronic Engineers on Industrial Electronics*, **38**, 4, 237–242.

LINKENS, D. A. and ABBOD, M., 1991, Self-organising fuzzy logic control for real-time processes, *Proceedings of Institution Electrical Engineers International Conference, Control 91*, Edinburgh, UK, **2**, 971–976, March.

LINKENS, D. A. and ABBOD, M. F., 1992, Self-organising fuzzy logic control and the selection of its scaling factors, *Transactions of the Institute of Measurement and Control*, **14**, 114–125.

LINKENS, D. A. and HASNAIN, S. B., 1991, Self-organising fuzzy logic control and its application to muscle relaxant anaesthesia, *Institution of Electrical Engineers Proceedings, Pt D, Control Theory and Applications*, **138**, 274–284.

LINKENS, D. A. and MAHFOUF, M., 1988, Knowledge elicitation of fuzzy logic control of drug infusion, Institution of Electrical Engineers Colloquium on Exploiting the Knowledge-base: Applications of Rule-based Control, London, UK, Digest No. 1989/89, pp. 3/1–3/3.

LINKENS, D. A. and MAHFOUF, M., 1994, Generalised predictive control (GPC) in clinical anaesthesia, in Clarke, D. W. (Ed), *Advances in Model-Based Predictive Control*, Oxford University Press, Oxford, UK, 429–445.

LINKENS, D. A. and NYONGESA, H. O., 1995, Genetic algorithms for fuzzy control. Part 1: offline system development and application, *Institution of Electrical Engineers Proceedings, Pt D, Control Theory and Applications*, **142**, 3, 161–176.

LINKENS, D. A., ASBURY, A. J. and BROWN, B. H., 1981, On-line control of muscle relaxant administration during anaesthesia, Institution of Electrical Engineers Conference on Control and its Applications, Warwick, UK.

LINKENS, D. A., GREENHOW, S. G. and ASBURY, A. J., 1990, Clinical trials with the anaesthetic expert adviser RESAC, Expert Systems in Medicine 6, London, UK, June, 11–18.

LINKENS, D. A., MAHFOUF, M. and ASBURY, A. J., 1991a, Multivariable Generalised Predictive Control for Anaesthesia, *Proceedings of First European Control Conference (ECC1)*, Grenoble, France, **2**, 1630–1635.

LINKENS, D. A., MAHFOUF, M. F. and ASBURY, A. J., 1991b, Generalised predictive control applied to muscle relaxant anaesthesia, IEE conference on adaptive control, Control 91, Edinburgh, UK, March, 790–794.

LINKENS, D. A., MENAD, M. and ASBURY, A. J., 1985, Smith predictor and self-tuning control of muscle relaxant drug administration, *Institute of Electrical Engineers Proceedings, Pt D, Control Theory and Applications*, **132**, 212–218.

LINKENS, D. A., ASBURY, A. J., RIMMER, S. J. and MENAD, M., 1982, Identification and control of muscle relaxant anaesthesia, *Institution of Electrical Engineers Proceedings, Pt D, Control Theory and Applications*, **129**, 136–141.

LJUNG, L., 1987, *System Identification: Theory for the User*, Prentice-Hall, Inc., Englewood Cliffs, New Jersey, USA.

LU, W. and FISHER, D. G., 1992, Non-minimal predictive control, *Chemical Engineering Sciences*, **47**, 4, 809–820.

MACLEOD, A. D., ASBURY, A. J., GRAY, W. M. and LINKENS, D. A., 1989, Automatic control of neuromuscular block with atracurium, *British Journal of Anaesthesia*, **63**, 31–35.

MAHFOUF, M., 1991, 'Adaptive control and identification for on-line drug infusion in anaesthesia', unpublished PhD thesis, Department of Automatic Control and Systems Engineering, University of Sheffield, UK.

MAHFOUF, M., LINKENS, D. A., ASBURY, A. J., GRAY, W. M. and PEACOCK, J. E., 1992, Generalised predictive control (GPC) in the operating theatre, *Institution of Electrical Engineers Proceedings, Pt D, Control Theory and Applications*, **139**, 5, 451–460.

MAITRE, P., VOZEH, S. and STANSKI, D., 1986, Correspondence letter, *Anaesthesiology*, **65**, 344–345.

MANSOUR, N. E. and LINKENS, D. A., 1988, Pole-assignment self-tuning control of blood pressure in postoperative patients: a simulation study, *Institute of Electrical Engineers Proceedings, Pt D, Control Theory and Applications*, **136**, 1–11.

MARSH, B., WHITE, M., NORTON, N. and KENNY, G. N. C., 1991, Pharmacokinetic model driven infusion of propofol in children, *British Journal of Anaesthesia*, **67**, 41–48.

MARSHALL, J. E., 1979, *Control of time-delay systems*, EE Control Engineering series 10, Peter Peregrinus Ltd, Stevenage, UK.

MCINTOSH, A. R., SHAH, S. L. and FISHER, D. G., 1989, Selection of tuning parameters for adaptive generalised predictive control, Proceedings of the American Control Conference, Pittsburg, 1828–1833.

MEAGER, A., LEUNG, H. and WOOLEY, J., 1989, Assays for tumor necrosis factor and related cytokines, *Journal of Immunological Methods*, **116**, 1–17.

MEIER, R., NIEUWLAND, J., ZBINDEN, A. M. and HACISALIHZADE, S. S., 1992, Fuzzy logic control of blood pressure during anaesthesia, *Institution of Electrical and Electronic Engineers Control Magazine*, 12–17.

MENAD, M., 1984, 'Feedback control of drug administration for muscle relaxation', unpublished PhD thesis, Department of Automatic Control and Systems Engineering, University of Sheffield, UK.

MILLARD, R. K., HUTTON, P., PEREIRA, E. and PRYS-ROBERTS, C., 1986, On using a self-tuning controller for blood pressure regulation during surgery, IMEKO Conference on Measurement in Clinical Medicine, Edinburgh, UK, 173–178.

MILLARD, R. K., MONK, C. R. and PRYS-ROBERTS, C., 1988a, Self-tuning control of hypotension during ENT surgery using a volatile anaesthetic, *Institution of Electrical Engineers Proceedings, Pt D, Control Theory and Applications*, **125**, 95–105.

MILLARD, R. K., MONK, C. R., WOODCOCK, T. E. and PRYS-ROBERTS, C., 1988b, Controlled hypotension during ENT surgery using self-tuners, *Biomedical Measurements Information and Control*, **2**, 2, 59–72.

MIZUMOTO, M., 1988, Fuzzy controls under various fuzzy reasoning methods, *International Journal of Man–Machine Studies*, **7**, 129–151.

MOHTADI, C., 1986, 'Studies in advanced self-tuning algorithms', unpublished DPhil. thesis, Oxford University, Oxford, UK.

MOHTADI, C., 1989, On the role of prefiltering in parameter estimation and control, in S. L. Shah and G. Dumont (Eds) *Lecture Notes in Control and Information Sciences*, Springer-

Verlag, 121–144.

MOHTADI, C., SHAH, S. L. and FISHER, D. G., 1992, Frequency response characteristics of MIMO GPC, *International Journal of Control*, **55**, 4, 877–900.

MOORE, C. G., 1991, 'Indirect adaptive fuzzy controllers', unpublished PhD thesis, Southampton University, Southampton, UK.

MORSHEDI, A. M., CUTLER, C. R. and SKEOVANEK, T. A., 1985, Optimal solution of dynamic matrix control with linear programming techniques (LDMC), American Control Conference, Boston, USA.

NIE, J. and LINKENS, D. A., 1995, *Fuzzy-Neural Control, Principles, Algorithms and Applications*, Prentice Hall, Hemel Hempstead, UK.

OLKKOLA, K. T. and SCHWILDEN, H., 1991, Use of a pharmacokinetic-dynamic model for the automatic feedback control of atracurium, *European Journal of Pharmacology*, **49**, 293–296.

OWENS, D. H., 1981, *Multivariable and Optimal Systems*, Academic Press, London, UK.

PATON, W. D. M. and WAUD, D. R., 1967, The margin of safety of neuromuscular blockade transmission, *Journal of Physiology (London)*, **191**, 59.

PEACOCK, J. E., LEWIS, R. P., REILLY, C. S. and NIMMO, W. S., 1990, Effect of different rates of infusion of propofol for induction of anaesthesia in elderly patients, *British Journal of Anaesthesia*, **65**, 436–352.

PRETT, D. M. and GILLETTE, R. D., 1980, Optimisation and constrained control of a catalytic cracking unit, Paper WP5-C, Proceedings of the Joint Automatic Control Conference, San Francisco, USA.

PROCYK, T. J., 1977, 'Self-organising control for dynamic processes', unpublished DPhil. thesis, Queen Mary College, London, UK.

PROCYK, T. J. and MAMDANI, E. H., 1979, Linguistic self-organising process controller, *Automatica*, **15**, 15–30.

RAMETTI, L. B., 1985, 'On-line control of d-tubocurarine-induced muscle relaxation', unpublished PhD thesis, University of Cape Town, South Africa.

RAMETTI, L. B., BRADLOW, H. S. and UYS, P. C., 1985, On-line parameter estimation and control of d-tubocurarine-induced muscle relaxation, *Medical Biology and Engineering Computation*, **23**, 556–564.

RAO, R. R., 1984, *Optimisation*, Wiley Eastern Limited, New Delhi, India.

RICHALET, J., RAULT, A., TESTUD, J. L. and PAPON, J., 1978, Model predictive heuristic control: applications to industrial processes, *Automatica*, **14**, 413–428.

ROBB, H. M., ASBURY, A. J., GRAY. W. M. and LINKENS, D. A., 1988, Towards automatic control of general anaesthesia, presentation at the conference 'Medical Informatics' 88, Nottingham, 121–126.

ROBB, H. M., ASBURY, A. J., GRAY, W. M. and LINKENS, D. A., 1993, Towards a standardised anaesthetic state using isoflurane and morphine, *British Journal of Anaesthesia*, **71**, 366–369.

ROBINSON, B. D. and CLARKE, D. W., 1991, Robustness effects of a prefilter in generalised predictive control, *Institution of Electrical Engineers Proceedings, Pt D, Control Theory and Applications*, **138**, 2–8.

SALZSIEDER, E., ALBRETCH, G., JUTZI, E. and FISCHER, U., 1984, Estimation of individually adapted control parameters for an artificial bera cell, *Biomedicia and Biochimica Acta*, **43**, 585–596.

SANCHEZ, J. M., 1995, *Adaptive Predictive Control – From Concept to Plant Optimisation*, Prentice Hall, Hemel Hempstead, UK.

SAVEGE, T. M., DUBOIS, M., FRANK, M. and HOLLY, J. M. P., 1978, Preliminary investigation into a new method of assessing the quality of anaesthesia: the cardiovascular response to a measured noxious stimulus, *British Journal of Anaesthesia*, **50**, 481–487.

SCHILLS, G. F., SASSE, F. G. and RIDEOUT, V. C., 1987, Automatic control of anaesthesia using two feedback variables, *Annals of Biomedical Engineering*, **15**, 19–34.

SCHUTTLER, J., SCHWILDEN, H. and STOECKEL, H., 1986, Pharmacokinetic-dynamic modeling of diprivan, *Anesthesiology*, **65**, A549.

SCHUTTLER, J., KLOOS, S., SCHWILDEN, H. and STOECKEL, H., 1988, Total intravenous anaesthesia with propofol and alfentanil by computer assisted infusion, *Anaesthesia (Supplement)*, **43**, 2–7.

SCHWILDEN, H., SCHUTTLER, J. and STOECKEL, H., 1987, Closed-loop feedback control of methohexital anaesthesia by quantitative EEG analysis in humans, *Anesthesiology*, **67**, 341–347.

SCHWILDEN, H., STOECKEL, H. and SCHUTTLER, J., 1989, Closed-loop feedback control of propofol anaesthesia by quantitative EEG analysis in humans, *British Journal of Anaesthesia*, **62**, 290–296.

SCOKAERT, P. O. M., 1994, 'Constrained predictive control', unpublished DPhil. thesis, University of Oxford, Oxford, UK.

SCOKAERT, P. O. M. and CLARKE, D. W., 1994, Stabilising properties of constrained predictive control, *Institution of Electrical Engineers Proceedings, Pt D, Control Theory and Applications*, **141**, 295–304.

SHAFER, A., 1995, STANPUMP, ftp://pkpd.icon.paloalto.med.va.gov/public/stanpump.dir/.

SHAFER, A., DOZE, V. A., SHAFER, S. and WHITE, P. F., 1988, Pharmacokinetics and pharmacodynamics of propofol infusions during general anaesthesia, *Anesthesiology*, **69**, 348–356.

SHEINER, L. B., ROSENBERG, B. and MELMON, K. L., 1972, Modelling of individual pharmacokinetics for computer-aided drug dosage, *Computers and Biomedical Research*, **5**, 441–459.

SHEINER, L. B., STANSKI, D. R., VOZEH, S., MILLER, R. D. and HAM, J., 1979, Simultaneous modelling of pharmacokinetics and pharmacodynamics: Application to d-tubocurarine, *Clinical Pharmacology and Therapeutics*, **25**, 358.

SHEPPARD, L. C., 1983, Guest editorial, *Medical Instrumentation*, **17**.

SHEPPARD, L. C., SHOTTS, J. F., ROBERSON, N. F., WALLACE, F. D. and KOUCHOUKOS, N. T., 1979, Simultaneous modelling of pharmacokinetics and pharmacodynamics: Application to d-Tubocurarine, *Clinical Pharmacology and Therapeutics*, **25**, 358.

SHOOK, D. S., MOHTADI, C. and SHAH, S. L., 1991, Identification for long-range predictive control, *Institution of Electrical Engineers Proceedings, Pt D, Control Theory and Applications*, **138**, 19, 75–84.

SHOOK, D. S., MOHTADI, C. and SHAH, S. L., 1992, A control-relevant identification strategy for GPC, *Transactions of the Institution of Electrical and Electronic Engineers on Automatic Control*, **137**, 7, 975–980.

SLATE, J. B., 1980, 'Model-based design of a controller for infusing sodium nitroprusside during post surgical hypertension', unpublished PhD thesis, University of Alabama, Birmingham, USA.

SLATE, J. B., SHEPPARD, L. C., RIDEOUT, V. C. and BLACKSTONE, E. H., 1979, A model for design of a blood pressure controller for hypertensive patients, 5th IFAC Symposium on Identification and Systems Parameter Estimation, Darmstadt, Germany.

SMITH, O. J. M., 1959, A controller to overcome dead-time, *Journal of the Instrument Society of America*, **6**, 23–33.

SMOLEN, V. F., TURRIE, B. D. and WIEGAND, W. A., 1972, Drug input optimisation: bioavailability-effected time optimal control of multiple simultaneous pharmacological effects and their interrelationships, *Journal of Pharmaceutical Sciences*, **61**, 1941–1952.

SOETERBOEK, R., 1992, *Predictive Control: A Unified Approach*, Prentice Hall International Series in Systems and Control Engineering, Hemel Hempstead, UK.

TACKLEY, R. M., LEWIS, G. T. R., PRYS-ROBERTS, C., BOADEN, R. W., DIXON, J. and HARVEY, J. T., 1989, Computer-controlled infusion of propofol, *British Journal of*

Anaesthesia, **62**, 46–53.

TATNALL, M. L., MORRIS, P. and WEST, P. G., 1981, Controlled anaesthesia: an approach using patients' characteristics identified during uptake, *British Journal of Anaesthesia*, **53**, 1019–1026.

TSANG, T. T. C. and CLARKE, D. W., 1988, Generalised predictive control with input constraints, *Institution of Electrical Engineers Proceedings, Pt D, Control Theory and Applications*, **135**, 6, 451–460.

TUFFS, P. S. and CLARKE, D. W., 1985, Self-tuning control of offset: a unified approach, *Institution of Electrical Engineers Proceedings, Pt D, Control Theory and Applications*, **132**, 100–110.

VAN DEN BOSCH, P. P. J., 1979, PSI: an extended interactive block oriented simulation program, IFAC Symposium on CAD Control Systems, 223–228.

VEALL, G. R. Q. and PEACOCK, J. E., 1994, Influence of circulation time on the onset of i.v. anaesthesia, *British Journal of Anaesthesia*, **73**, 272P.

VOZEH, S. and STEIMER, J. L., 1985, Feedback control methods for drug dosage optimization, *Clinical Pharmacokinetics*, **10**, 457–476.

WAIT, C. M., GOAT, V. A. and BLOGG, C. E., 1987, Feedback control of neuromuscular blockade. A simple system for infusion of atracurium, *Anaesthesia*, **42**, 1212–1217.

WARD, S., NEILL, E. A. M., WEATHERLEY, B. C. and CORALL, I. M., 1983, Pharmacokinetics of Atracurium Besylate in healthy patients (after a single i.v. bolus dose), *British Journal of Anaesthesia*, **55**, 113.

WARWICK, K., ZHU, Q. M. and DOUCE, J. L., 1991, An adaptive controller for nonlinear systems, *Preprints of the IEE Conference on adaptive controllers*, Herriot-Watt University, Edinburgh, UK, 651–656.

WAUD, D. R. and WAUD, B. E., 1971, The relation between tetanic fade and receptor occlusion in the presence of competitive neuromuscular block, *Anesthesiology*, **35**, 456.

WEATHERLEY, B. C., WILLIAMS, S. G. and NEIL, E. A. M., 1983, Pharmacokinetics, pharmacodynamics and dose response relationship of Atracurium administered i.v., *British Journal of Anaesthesia*, **55**, 39S.

WEBSTER, N. R. and COHEN, A. T., 1987, Closed-loop administration of Atracurium. Steady-state neuromuscular blockade during surgery using a computer controlled closed-loop Atracurium infusion, *Anaesthesia*, **42**, 1085–1091.

WELLSTEAD, P. E., 1980, 'Self-tuning control systems: the pole-zero assignment approach', SERC vacation school on computer control, University of Sheffield, UK, September, 9.1–9.34.

WELLSTEAD, P. E. and GALE, S., 1978, Self-tuning pole/zero assignment predictions, Control Systems Centre, Report No. 412, UMIST, Manchester, UK.

WELLSTEAD, P. E., PRAGER, D., ZANKER, P. and EDMUNDS, J. M., 1978, Self-tuning pole/zero regulators, Control Systems Centre, Report No. 404, UMIST, Manchester, UK.

WHITE, M. and KENNY, G. N. C., 1990, Intravenous propofol anaesthesia using a computerised infusion system, *Anaesthesia*, **45**, 204–209.

WHITING, B. and KELMAN. A. W., 1980, The modelling of drug response, *Clinical Science*, **59**, 311–314.

WILKINSON, D. J., MORRIS, A. J. and THAM, M. T., 1994, Multivariable constrained predictive control (with application to high performance distillation), *International Journal of Control*, **59**, 841–862.

WITTENMARK, B., MIDDLETON, R. H. and GOODWIN, G. C., 1987, Adaptive decoupling of multivariable systems, *International Journal of Control*, **46**, 6, 1993–2009.

YDSTIE, B. E., 1984, Extended horizon adaptive control, IFAC Proceedings of the 9th Triennal World Congress, Budapest, Hungary, 911–915.

YOON, T. W. and CLARKE, D. W., 1994, Towards robust adaptive predictive control, in Clarke, D. W. (Ed.) *Advances in Model-based Predictive Control*, Oxford University

Press, Oxford, UK.

ZADEH, L. A., 1965, Fuzzy sets, *Information and Control*, **12**, 94–102.

ZADEH, L. A., 1973, An outline of a new approach to the analysis of complex systems and decision processes, *Transactions of the Institution of Electrical and Electronic Engineers on Automatic Control*, **SMC-3**, 28–44.

ZHANG, L. and CAMERON, R. G., 1989, A real-time expert control strategy for blood gas management in neonates under ventilation treatment, Institution of Electrical Engineers Colloquium on Exploiting the Knowledge-base: Applications of Rule-based Control, Digest No. 1989/89, London, UK, 4/1–4/7.

ZIEGLER, J. G. and NICHOLS, N. B., 1942, Optimum settings for automatic controllers, *Transactions of the American Society of Mechanical Engineers*, **64**, 759.

Index

T - #0052 - 071024 - C0 - 254/178/16 [18] - CB - 9780748405978 - Gloss Lamination